Conventional and Powder Mixed Electro-Discharge Machining

This book presents the evolution of the electro-discharge machining (EDM) process from conventional EDM to powder mixed EDM with emphases on biomedical applications. It discusses the theory behind each process and their applications in the field of biomedical research, and presents a brief background to various EDM processes, current research challenges, and detailed case studies of powder mixed EDM of various materials. It also includes a state-of-the-art review of the EDM process.

Features:

- Focuses on biomedical implant and device manufacturing using commercialization of powder mixed electro-discharge machining (PM-EDM) technology.
- Discusses surface modification of biomaterials through the PM-EDM process.
- Reviews processing of the metallic biomaterials for biomedical applications.
- Explores optimization of the process factors for achieving optimal responses using NSGA-II.
- Includes comprehensive mechanism and application details of the PM-EDM process.

This book is aimed at graduate students and researchers in manufacturing, production, materials, and biomedical engineering.

Advances in Design, Materials and Manufacturing for Sustainability
Series Editors: Jitendra Kumar Katiyar and T V V L N Rao

Conventional and Powder Mixed Electro-Discharge Machining
Biomedical Applications
Edited by Ahmad Majdi Abdul-Rani, Masdi Muhammad, T V V L N Rao,
Saeed Rubaiee, Anas Ahmed, and Mohd Danish

For more information about this series, please visit: www.routledge.com/Advances-in-Design-Materials-and-Manufacturing-for-Sustainability/book-series/CRCADMMS

Conventional and Powder Mixed Electro-Discharge Machining

Biomedical Applications

Edited by
Ahmad Majdi Abdul-Rani, Masdi Muhammad,
T V V L N Rao, Saeed Rubaiee, Anas Ahmed, and
Mohd Danish

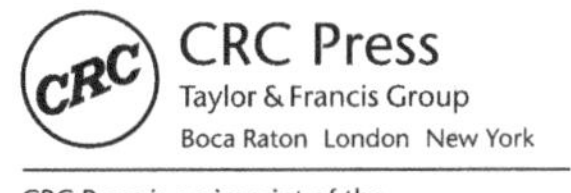

CRC Press
Taylor & Francis Group
Boca Raton London New York

CRC Press is an imprint of the
Taylor & Francis Group, an **informa** business

Designed cover image: Shutterstock

First edition published 2025
by CRC Press
2385 NW Executive Center Drive, Suite 320, Boca Raton FL 33431

and by CRC Press
4 Park Square, Milton Park, Abingdon, Oxon, OX14 4RN

CRC Press is an imprint of Taylor & Francis Group, LLC

ISBN: 9781032452760 (hbk)
ISBN: 9781032597300 (pbk)
ISBN: 9781003456018 (ebk)

DOI: 10.1201/9781003456018

Typeset in Times
by Newgen Publishing UK

Contents

Alexis Mouangue Nanimina, Ahmad Majdi Abdul-Rani,
Elhuseini Garba, and Saeed Rubaiee

Chapter 3   Surface Analysis of Magnesium Alloy Processed Using
C-EDM and PM-EDM Method 83

*Muhammad Al'Hapis Abdul Razak, Ahmad Majdi Abdul-Rani,
Iqtidar Ahmed Gul, Elhuseini Garba, Syed Shehzeb Abdullah, and
Anas Ahmed*

Chapter 4   Innovative Biomimetic Electro-Discharge Coating on
Bulk Metallic Glass for Potential Orthopedic Application 100

*Abdul Azeez Abdu Aliyu, Ahmad Majdi Abdul-Rani, Iqtidar Ahmed
Gul, Elhuseini Garba, Tang Tong Boon, Nabihah Bt Sallih, and
Sadaqat Ali*

Chapter 5   Material Transfer Rate During Electro-Discharge Process: Modeling and Optimization 109

Abdul Azeez Abdu Aliyu, Ahmad Majdi Abdul-Rani, Iqtidar Ahmed Gul, Muhammad Usman, Boonrat Lohwongwatana, and Ahmad Nasiru Hamza

Chapter 6   Arc Discharge Method for Aluminium Oxide Nanoparticle Synthesis 124

Shahruzaman Sulaiman, Ahmad Majdi Abdul-Rani, T V V L N Rao, Mohd Danish, and Maysarah Binti Al-Amin

xi

Foreword

Adaptation of technological advancement is crucial for companies to survive in the environment of cutting-edge competitors. I am extremely delighted that my enthusiastic academic collaborator, Dr Ahmad Majdi Abdul Rani has attempted to write a book on the up-gradation of Electric Discharge Machining for biomedical applications.

This book will reveal the innovative opportunity for the industrialists to employ the working operation of Electric Discharge Machining for fabrication and coating process simultaneously. The commercialization of this concept will provide a cost-effective solution for precise productivity as well as the biocompatibility of end-products.

I compliment Dr Ahmad Majdi and his team for putting this tremendous effort into book publication and looking forward to reading the contents of the book.

Izhar Abd Aziz

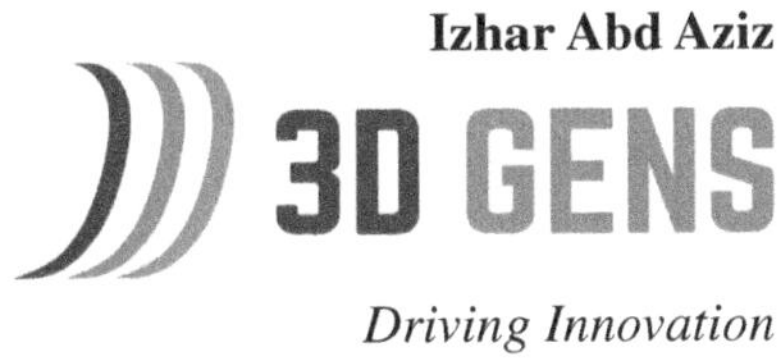

Driving Innovation

Preface

The experience in the form of information must be transferred to the subsequent generations to furnish a research platform for continual improvement in society.

After acquiring the achievements of patent filing, conference awards, and high impact factor journal publications in the research area of powder mixed electric discharge machining (PM-EDM) and its utilization in biomedical applications, an idea hit my mind to bestow my knowledge and experience in the form of a book to the audience. The book focuses on the surface modification of commonly used metallic biomaterials through an emerging technique of PM-EDM. The scope of the book includes novel technological advancements of PM-EDM in the field of metallic biomaterials. The chapters highlight the innovative ways of mechanical experimentation and metallurgical characterization towards biomedical applications. It opens up a window of opportunity for professional industrialists to commercialize the technology of PM-EDM for biomedical implants and devices.

Ahmad Majdi Abdul-Rani, Masdi Muhammad,
T V V L N Rao, Saeed Rubaiee,
Anas Ahmed, and Mohd Danish
Editors, Conventional and Powder
Mixed Electro-Discharge Machining

About the Editors

Ahmad Majdi Abdul-Rani has a PhD in Mechanical Engineering from Loughborough University. His research interests include biomedical engineering, additive manufacturing, and reverse engineering. He heads the Advanced Biomedical Materials and Manufacturing group at Universiti Teknologi PETRONAS. He is Vice-Chairman of the American Society of Mechanical Engineers (Malaysian Chapter) and a member of ASME International, the Society of Manufacturing Engineers, and the Malaysian Society for Engineering and Technology. He recently received the U.K.'s Leadership in Innovation Fellowship Newton Award. He has three patents, over 150 publications, and has secured several research grants. He has been with the Mechanical Engineering Department at Universiti Teknologi PETRONAS since 1998, previously serving as Head from 2009 to 2011. He has supervised over 20 postgraduate students.

Masdi Muhammad chairs the Mechanical Engineering Department at Universiti Teknologi PETRONAS. He holds a BSc and MSc in Mechanical Engineering from Lehigh University and a PhD in Mechanical Engineering from UTP, researching reliability modeling for multi-state degradation systems. His research interests include reliability and maintenance. He has over seven postgraduate students and is actively involved in research, consultancy, and training. Before joining UTP, he worked for 12 years in process and equipment engineering, product development, and material quality at Malaysia's leading U.S. semiconductor company. He is a chartered engineer, certified reliability engineer, certified maintenance and reliability professional, and member of several professional societies. He also holds a certification in project leadership.

T V V L N Rao is Dean of the Faculty of Engineering at Assam Down Town University. He received his PhD in Tribology from IIT Delhi and MTech in Mechanical Manufacturing from NIT Calicut. His research interests include tribology, lubrication, bearings, machining, and manufacturing. He has authored over 140 publications and secured several research grants. Rao serves as an editor and reviewer for various tribology journals. He is a member of the Malaysian Tribology Society, Society of Tribologists and Lubrication Engineers, and Tribology Society of India. He has previously held positions at SRMIST, LNMIIT, Universiti Teknologi PETRONAS, and BITS Pilani. Throughout his career, he has made significant contributions to the field of tribology through his research, publications, and service.

Saeed Rubaiee received his BS in Chemical Engineering from Tennessee Tech University, MSc in Industrial Engineering from the University of South Florida, and PhD from the Department of Industrial and Manufacturing Engineering at Wichita State University. He is an Associate Professor in the Department of Industrial and Systems Engineering at the University of Jeddah in Saudi Arabia. His research interests include engineering systems, sustainability, manufacturing engineering, renewable energy, advanced materials, and applied optimization. He has published extensively in high-impact factor journals. Throughout his career, Dr Rubaiee has contributed significant industrial and manufacturing engineering research.

Anas Ahmed received his BS in Electrical Engineering and MSc in Electrical and Computer Engineering from the University of Miami. He completed an MSc in Industrial Engineering and PhD in Industrial Engineering from the University of Miami. He is currently an Associate Professor in the Department of Industrial and Systems Engineering at the University of Jeddah in Saudi Arabia. His diverse research interests include game theory, optimization, logistics, materials engineering, energy, disaster management, and statistical quality control. Dr Ahmed has contributed high-impact research across various fields throughout his career by publishing in reputable journals.

Mohd Danish received his BS and MSc in Mechanical Engineering from Aligarh Muslim University in India. He completed his PhD in Mechanical Engineering from Universiti Teknologi PETRONAS in Malaysia. Dr Danish is an Assistant Professor in the Department of Mechanical and Materials Engineering at the University of Jeddah. His research interests include sustainable and cryogenic machining, hybrid machining, EDM, 3D printing, SLM, and multi-objective optimization. He has published extensively in high-impact journals, making significant contributions to mechanical engineering through his research.

Contributors

Abdul Azeez Abdu Aliyu
Department of Mechanical Engineering, Bayero University Kano, Nigeria

Ahmad Majdi Abdul-Rani
Universiti Teknologi PETRONAS, Department of Mechanical Engineering, Perak, Malaysia

Muhammad Al'Hapis Abdul Razak
Manufacturing Section, Universiti Kuala Lumpur Malaysian Spanish Institute, Malaysia

Syed Shehzeb Abdullah
Department of Mechanical Engineering, Capital University of Science & Technology, Islamabad, Pakistan

Azlan Ahmad
Universiti Teknologi PETRONAS, Department of Mechanical Engineering, Perak, Malaysia

Habib Ahmad
Department of Mechanical Engineering, Pakistan Institute of Engineering and Applied Sciences, Pakistan

Anas Ahmed
Department of Industrial and System Engineering, University of Jeddah, Jeddah, Saudi Arabia

Maysarah Binti Al-Amin
Universiti Teknologi PETRONAS, Department of Mechanical Engineering, Perak, Malaysia

Md Al-Amin
School of Mechanical and Mining Engineering, The University of Queensland, St Lucia, Australia

Sadaqat Ali
National University of Sciences and Technology (NUST), Islamabad, Pakistan

Tang Tong Boon
Institute of Health and Analytics (IHA), University Technology PETRONAS, Perak, Malaysia

Mohd Danish
Department of Mechanical and Materials Engineering, University of Jeddah, Jeddah, Saudi Arabia

Elhuseini Garba
Universiti Teknologi PETRONAS, Department of Mechanical Engineering, Perak, Malaysia

Iqtidar Ahmed Gul
Universiti Teknologi PETRONAS, Department of Mechanical Engineering, Perak, Malaysia

Ahmad Nasiru Hamza
Department of Electrical Engineering, Kano University of Science and Technology, Wudil

Nor Liyana Safura Hashim
Department of Biomedical Engineering and Health Sciences, Faculty of Electrical Engg., Universiti Teknologi Malaysia

Adeel Hassan
Universiti Teknologi PETRONAS, Department of Mechanical Engineering, Perak, Malaysia

Nor Hisham Khamis
Department of Communication
 Engineering, Faculty of Electrical
 Engineering, Universiti Teknologi
 Malaysia

Boonrat Lohwongwatana
Department of Metallurgical
 Engineering, Faculty of Engineering,
 Chulalongkorn University, Bangkok,
 Thailand

Nazriah Mahmud
Department of Biomedical Engineering
 and Health Sciences, Universiti
 Teknologi Malaysia

Alexis Mouangue Nanimina
Mechanical Engineering Department,
 Higher National Institute of Sciences
 and Techniques of Abéché, Abéché,
 Chad

Kartiko Nugroho
Department of Biomedical Engineering
 and Health Sciences, Universiti
 Teknologi Malaysia

T V V L N Rao
Faculty of Engineering, Assam
 down town University, Guwahati,
 Assam, India

Saeed Rubaiee
Department of Mechanical and
 Materials Engineering, University of
 Jeddah, Saudi Arabia

Nabihah Bt Sallih
Institute of Health and Analytics (IHA),
 University Technology PETRONAS,
 Perak, Malaysia

Shahruzaman Sulaiman
Manufacturing Section, Universiti
 Kuala Lumpur Kampus Cawangan
 Malaysian Spanish Institute

Muhammad Usman
Department of Aeronautics &
 Astronautics, Institute of Space
 Technology (IST), Islamabad,
 Pakistan

Azli Yahya
Department of Electronic and Computer
 Engineering, Faculty of Electrical
 Engineering, Universiti Teknologi
 Malaysia

1 Conventional EDM of Titanium and Molybdenum Alloys

Alexis Mouangue Nanimina, Ahmad Majdi Abdul-Rani, Masdi Muhammad, T V V L N Rao, and Elhuseini Garba

1.1 INTRODUCTION

Die-sinker electro-discharge machining (EDM) represented in Figure 1.1 is a repeated battering of electrode against a workpiece. The tool is the reverse shape of the part to be machined. Die-sinker EDM is traditionally performed vertically, but could also be applied horizontally [1]. In die-sinker EDM machines, the electrode and workpiece are submersed in dielectric fluid during the machining process. The electrode is lowered down by servo control to a few millimeters from the workpiece. Die-sinker EDM machine can produce complex cavities out of a workpiece. Die-sinker EDM machines vary in sizes and operating mode, from manual operating table system to large automatic computer numerical control (CNC) [1]. The main sub-systems of die-sinker EDM are power supply, dielectric fluid, servo system, and electrode.

1.2 EDM WORKING PRINCIPLE

The material removing mechanism employed in EDM is by repeating the flow of sparks between the electrode and workpiece. The DC power supply is usually between 20 and 300 V with several milli-amperes of peak current applied to the workpiece and electrode, both of which are placed in a dielectric fluid. The dielectric fluid acts as an insulator to transient electrical discharge. In EDM, the mechanism of material removal is based on a series of erosion effects and theories, such as electro-mechanical, thermo-mechanical, and thermo-electrical. When a voltage is supplied between an electrode and a workpiece, the machining process undergoes five steps as shown in Figure 1.2.

Step 1: Voltage is applied between the electrode and workpiece creating an electric. As a result of the electric field, free electrons are emitted from the electrode and accelerated under electrostatic force towards the workpiece. At the end of Step 1, the voltage decreases while electric current is established between the electrode and workpiece as the dielectric fluid becomes a localized conductor.

DOI: 10.1201/9781003456018-1

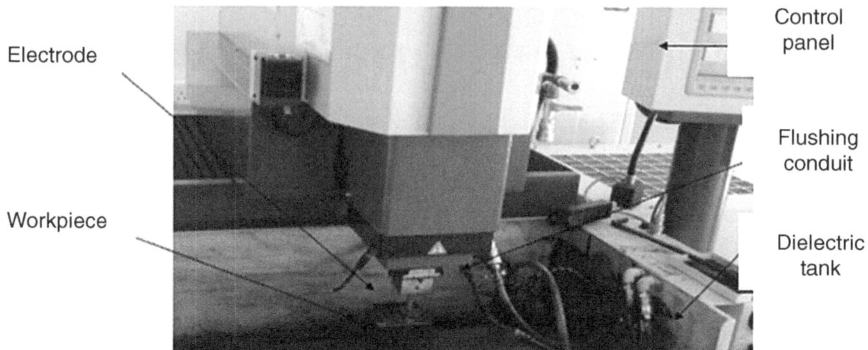

FIGURE 1.1 Die-sinker EDM machine EA8.

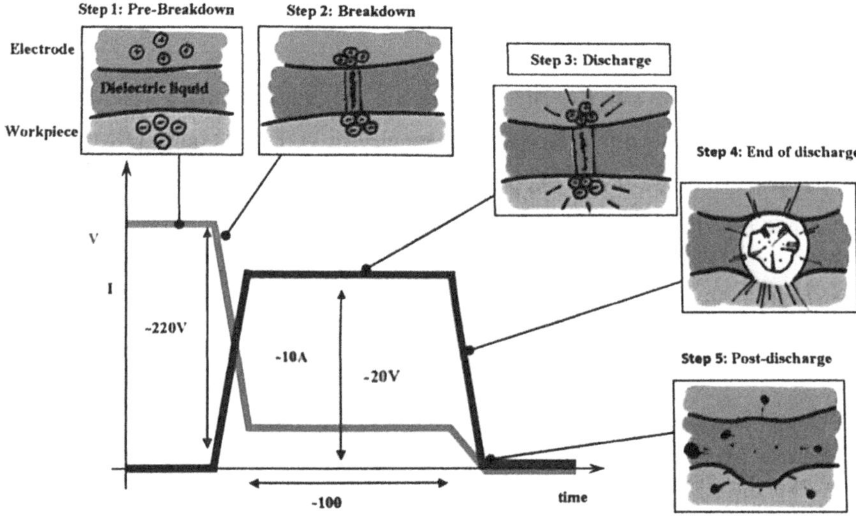

FIGURE 1.2 Principle of the EDM process.

Step 2: The emitted electrons hit the molecules of the dielectric fluid. Consequently, the dielectric fluid molecules become ionized if the energy of electrons is sufficient. Dielectric fluid becomes locally an electric conductor under the electrode and workpiece zone. Many electrons and ions will flow between the electrode and workpiece.

Step 3: The concentration of electrons becomes so much that it forms plasma of electrical discharges and will be seen in channel as a bright light of spark. Accelerated electrons and ions impact the surface of the electrode and workpiece and convert them into thermal energy. Intense localized heat flux leads to extreme instantaneous rise in temperature between 8000 and 12,000°C [2]. This melts, vaporizes, and removes the material.

Step 4: Upon withdrawal of potential difference, plasma channel collapses. This ultimately creates compression shock waves on both the electrode surfaces.

Step 5: Expelled molten material forms a crater around the zone of spark. The whole sequence of operation occurs within a few seconds from the start of the cycle. Machining parameters affecting the EDM output results such as material removal rate (MRR), surface roughness, and surface morphology are electric current, voltage, ON-time since the electrical discharge energy, E_e, and discharge heat q. These parameters are related as shown in equations (1.1) and (1.2).

$$E = U_e I_e t_i \tag{1.1}$$

where: U_e: discharge voltage, I_e: discharge current, t_i: ON-time.

$$q_e \cong \frac{U_e . I_e}{r_e^2 \pi} \tag{1.2}$$

where: r_e is the discharge radius.

1.3 COMPONENTS OF EDM SYSTEM

The basic EDM components are described in this section.

1.3.1 DIELECTRIC FLUIDS

Dielectric fluid is a medium used in EDM as insulator between a workpiece and an electrode. Under the effect of electric field due to applied voltage between the electrode and workpiece, the dielectric fluid is ionized and becomes a localized conductor where sparks are concentrated. The dielectric fluid regains the gap condition after discharge, cools the electrode and workpiece, and flushes away the debris from machining. The two commonly used dielectric fluids are petroleum-based hydrocarbon mineral oils and deionized water. The main properties of dielectric are high flush points and the viscosities. High insulation, high density, and high viscosity dielectric have positive effects on spark concentration [3]. Increasing the dielectric fluid pressure will reduce the surface roughness. The flushing is to clean the debris from the gap between the electrode and workpiece, and consequently improve the rate of material removal [4]. One of the main roles of dielectric fluid is to prevent oxidation which can lead to flaming. Oxidation is undesirable since it leads to oxide burning, which reduces surface electrical conductivity and, thereby, affects the machining process.

1.3.2 ELECTRODE MATERIALS

In die-sinker EDM, the electrode is used for relaying the sparks to the workpiece to remove materials. Different types of electrode materials are used, and these have respective effects on the product. Some electrode materials remove the materials efficiently but have high wear, while others have slight wear but remove the materials slowly [5]. The basic requirements for selecting electrode material are: high electrical conductivity to promote more electrons since electric current is the "cutting tool"; high melting point for better wear ratio since EDM is a thermal process and high thermal conductivity to quickly dissipate the heat from the EDM process through the electrode. The above properties determine the electrode spark-resisting capability of an electrode. Electrode materials should be fabricated easily with reasonable cost. The most used electrode materials include graphite, copper, bronze copper–tungsten (Cu–W), tungsten, and brass [6]. Selection of electrode material in die-sinker EDM should be a key decision before any experimental plan.

1.3.3 POWER SYSTEM

EDM power system transforms the alternative current (AC) power into pulsed direct current (DC) power with 30–300 V and several milli-ampere of peak current. The power system produces DC discharge current which flows between the electrode and workpiece. It also controls other electrical parameters such as voltage, frequency, and electrode polarity. A capacitor placed in the power system stores electricity through a resistor and discharges it on the workpiece through the electrode. The time at which the capacitor is being charged is the OFF-time and the discharging time is ON-time. The power system generates and supplies power into the dielectric fluid in the discharge gap. There are different types of EDM power generators that can store energy in an intermediate storage (capacitance) and discharge it as an electrical energy into a load in a single short pulse. These include the RC-type generator, rotary impulse trigger generator, electronic pulse generator, and hybrid EDM generator. The power system can generate and supply the power into the dielectric fluid in the discharge gap. There are different types of EDM power generators that can store energy in an intermediate storage (capacitance) and discharge it as an electrical energy into a load in a single short pulse. These include the RC-type generator, rotary impulse trigger generator, electronic pulse generator, and hybrid EDM generator.

1.3.4 SERVO CONTROL SYSTEM

The servo control system is used to keep the inter-electrode gap within a small distance during machining process. The gap size control is vital in EDM machining because it maintains efficient spark [7]. The requirements for an EDM servo control system are: electrode must not touch the workpiece, the electrode must advance toward and retract from the workpiece to maintain the voltage between the electrode and workpiece.

1.4 EDM APPLICATION AND LIMITATION

EDM process uses high energy for electric–thermal erosion (instead of mechanical cutting forces) to remove the material. Thus, EDM can machine "difficult-to-cut" materials such as titanium alloy, hard steels, carbides, and diamond. Besides, EDM is effective in machining brittle electrically conductive materials since no direct contact between the electrode and workpiece, thus no significant mechanical force is employed on the workpiece. EDM can machine complicated shapes with prefabricated tools. The process is particularly well suited to producing cavities and drilling irregular (complex) shaped holes.

EDM process is limited to electrically conductive workpiece materials. The workpiece conductivity of 0.1 ($\Omega^{-1}Cm^{-1}$) is considered as the minimum value for EDM to be effective. Other limitations of EDM include electrode wear and irregularity of the electrode wear. Also, EDM can only be used to machine sharp corners because of the existing gap between the electrode and workpiece. The surface layers of workpiece machined by EDM may be altered metallurgically and chemically due to the extremely high thermal energy process (up to 12,000°C) accompanied by the dielectric cooling process. The surface layer usually differs significantly from the base in the metallurgical structures due to recasting and contains gas holes, tool material particles, and other impurities from the dielectric fluid.

1.5 EDM RECENT WORKS

Research in conventional EDM includes improving the performance measures, such as MRR, surface quality, monitoring, and controlling of the process, such as pulse/ time and frequency, EDM developments, such as electrode design and manufacture; and optimizing the process variables. Table 1.1 presents some research finding in conventional EDM. Other research on the EDM process has been performed using different types of workpiece materials and various machining conditions. Results

TABLE 1.1
Research on conventional EDM

Authors/ Reference	Work material/ electrode	Output measures	Remarks
Hasçalık and Çaydaş (2007) [13]	Ti–6Al–4V/ graphite and aluminum	Surface topography, crack, Ra, MRR	Optimal set of machining parameters, such as peak current and ON and OFF-times was identified.
Kiyak and Çakır (2007) [14]	Tool steel/rod pure copper	Workpiece surface finish quality, surface roughness of electrode	Ra increased with increasing peak current and ON-time. Trends of Ra of workpiece and electrode are similar with same machining conditions.
Guu et al. (2001, 2007) [15, 16]	D2 Tool steel, Fe-Mn-Al alloy/ copper	Ra, recast layer, tensile strength, machining damage	Recast layer is thicker with high IP ON-time. Good, machined finish and reduces tensile residual stress obtained at low pulse energy. The EDM process induces damage on the machined surface.
Chrisna et al. (2008) [17]	Maraging steel/ copper	MRR, Ra, hardness	MRR increases with increases in current. Ra increases with increases in current. When current increases, hardness decreases. Crack widths increased due to the high temperature.

have shown that the effects of EDM occur on any type of workpiece material. The Ra, MRR, EWR, and overcut vary due to changes in the EDM parameters [8]. Overall, conventional EDM shows some advantages and disadvantages. The increase in the EDM machining parameters that induce a rough machined surface is seen as a disadvantage in terms of EDM performance, but it is an advantage in biomedical applications in terms of the implant surface or osseointegration.

1.6 EDM ON TITANIUM ALLOY IMPLANTS

In EDM of implants, a high set of peak current, voltage, and ON-time in EDM induces a sufficient macro-surface and creates a carbon enriched surface layer for improvement of osseointegration. It has been shown that EDM causes chemical and mechanical changes to the machined surface such as surface texture, hardness, and fatigue performance. Since during the EDM process, material is heated, melted, and cooled down by dielectric fluid to be resolidified thus, EDM is considered as a surface treatment process required for improvement of osseointegration. The limitation in using EDM as potential machining of implants is the fatigue performance [9]. Starsky et al. [10] and Manivasagam et al. [11] during their EDM research found that poor fatigue is due to the hardness effect of titanium alloys. Chen et al. [12] found that EDM is useful for modification and improvement of implant surfaces. In EDM, the resulting machined surface properties are mostly dependent on input ON-time, peak current, gap voltage thus, the quantity and duration of thermal energy hitting the workpiece surface.

1.7 METHODOLOGY

Design of experiment (DOE) is a statistical method used to plan, conduct, analyze, and interpret controlled experiments to evaluate the factors that control the value of a parameter or group of parameters.

1.8 DESIGN OF EXPERIMENT

A DOE was done and response surface methodology (RSM) techniques were selected using central composite design (CCD) which has the advantage that certain level adjustments are acceptable. Figure 1.5 presents the flow of DOE procedures. RSM was selected as design technique for this research since the electrical discharge machining process involves many machining parameters. Some machining parameters have interaction effects on output responses. As stated earlier, RSM could analyze the individual and interaction effects of the machining parameters on the responses, and it can predict the most important parameter according to analysis of variance (ANOVA). Depending on where the star points are placed, there are three types of CCD in RSM such as circumscribed CCD (CCC), inscribed CCD (CCI), and face-centered CCD (CCF). In CCC, the star points are at some distance alpha (α) from the center based on the properties desired for the design and the number of factors in the design. The star points establish new extremes for the low and high settings for all factors. Whereas in CCI, the design uses the factor settings as the star points and creates a factorial or fractional factorial design within those limits (in other words, a CCI design is a scaled-down CCC design with each factor level of the CCC design divided by α to generate the CCI design). This design also requires five levels of each factor. For CCF design, the star points are at the center of each face of the factorial space, so α = ± 1. This variety requires three levels of each factor.

1.9 PARAMETERS

1.9.1 Specimens

Titanium alloy Ti-6Al-4V grade 5 according to ASTM designation B.265-79 and molybdenum high-speed steel specifically, SKH51 according to Japanese industrial Standards (JIS) designation were selected as the workpiece materials. For the specimen preparation, CNC EDM Wire-cut machine FA10 brand was used to cut the raw material into block shape required for clamping on EDM. Titanium alloys and molybdenum high-speed steel specimens were prepared to the size of 9 mm × 11 mm × 5 mm for ease of mounting on analysis device requirement. Table 1.2 and Table 1.3 present, respectively, the chemical compositions of titanium alloy and molybdenum high-speed steel materials. The properties of the workpiece materials are presented in Table 1.4.

TABLE 1.2
Composition of molybdenum high-speed steel

Elements	C	Si	Cr	V	W	Mo	Co	Fe
Weight (%)	0.83	0.35	3.75	1.18	1.75	8.70	–	Balance

TABLE 1.3
Composition of titanium alloy

Elements	Al	V	Fe	O	C	N	H	Ti
Weight (%)	5.5–6.75	3.5–4.5	≤0.40	≤0.20	≤0.080	≤0.050	≤0.015	87.6–91

TABLE 1.4
Properties of workpiece materials

Materials	Melting point (°C)	Density (g/cm³)	Young modulus GPa	Thermal conductivity W/m.K	Hardness (HB)	Electrical resistivity x10⁻⁷Ωm
Molybdenum high-speed steel	1082.0	7.72–8	190–210	19.0	111.0	0.6
Titanium alloy	1660	4.43	120	7.3	334	7.36

TABLE 1.5
Copper–tungsten (W70Cu30) properties

Material	Melting point (°C)	Density (g/cm³)	Young modulus (N/mm²)	Hardness (HV)	Thermal conductivity (W/mK)	Electrical resistivity ×10⁻⁷ Ωcm
W70Cu30	3410	14.3	225×10^3	175	154	7.27

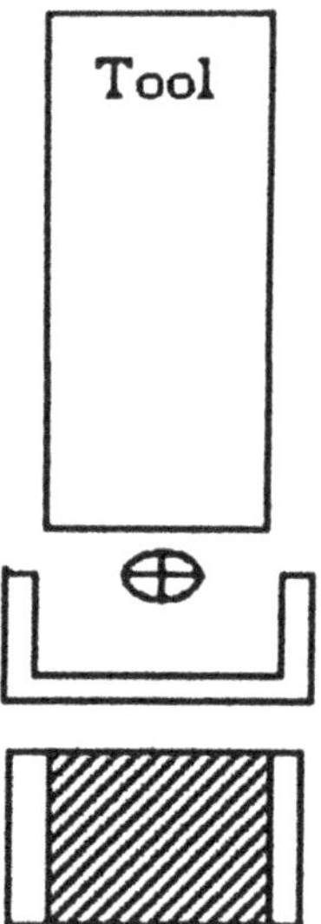

FIGURE 1.3   Cross-section of electrode position and workpiece U shape.

1.9.2   ELECTRODE MATERIAL

Cu–W (W70Cu30) was used as electrode material with cross-section of 9 mm × 9 mm. The selection of Cu–W is due to good conductivity of copper and good melting point of tungsten. High electrical conductivity of electrode promotes more electrons from electrode since electric current is the "cutting tool" and high melting point of electrode contributes low wear ratio since EDM is a thermal process. The combination of Cu–W gives optimal electrical and thermal conductivities to the electrode. Table 1.5 presents copper and Cu–W properties.

A square section 9 mm × 9 mm of electrodes was to machine a U-shape workpiece as shown in Figure 1.3.

1.10   EXPERIMENTS

The summary of the different categories of experiments is presented in Table 1.6.

TABLE 1.6
Different categories of experiments

No	Experiments	Category
1	**Experiment 1**	Conventional EDM on Ti-4Al-6V grade 5 titanium alloy
2	**Experiment 2**	Conventional EDM of molybdenum high-speed steel SKH51

Experiment 1: In Experiment 2, EDM on machining Ti-4Al-6V grade 5 titanium alloy was conducted without nano aluminum and nano tungsten.

Experiment 2: For experiment 3, EDM on molybdenum high-speed steel SKH51 without any metallic powders.

1.10.1 Output Responses

The output responses investigated in this research such as surface roughness, surface morphology, phase analysis, micro-hardness, fatigue performance, MRR, electrode wear ratio (EWR), and radial overcut (ROC) are presented and described as follows.

1.10.2 Surface Roughness Measurement

Surface roughness average (Ra), defined in ASME B46.1-2002 [18], was selected. Measurements were performed on all samples using surface roughness tester presented in Figure 1.4.

Ra is an important parameter used in manufacturing to measure the texture of machined surface which characterizes the quality of the machined surface of a product. Part that has good Ra improves the fatigue performance and corrosion resistance. However, roughness of biomedical implants can contribute to adhesion between the implant and a living bone [19], with rougher surface providing better adhesion but can be detrimental towards resistance to corrosion and fatigue. Craters, voids, and micro-cracks on implant surface reduce their fatigue and corrosion resistance. The measurements were done according to standard ISO 3274:1996 for the nominal characteristics of contact (Stylus) instruments. Three different measurement lines were taken and an average calculated. The stylus traverses the surface peaks and valleys, and the vertical motion of the stylus is converted by the transducer into an electrical signal which will be analyzed by digital or analog technique. The result in digital profile is stored in a computer and can be analyzed. Sample length was 6 mm, and the cut-off length was 2.5 mm.

1.10.3 Material Removal Rate

MRR is an important parameter selected to estimate the volume of material removed during a specific time of EDM machining process. MRR is a parameter that describes

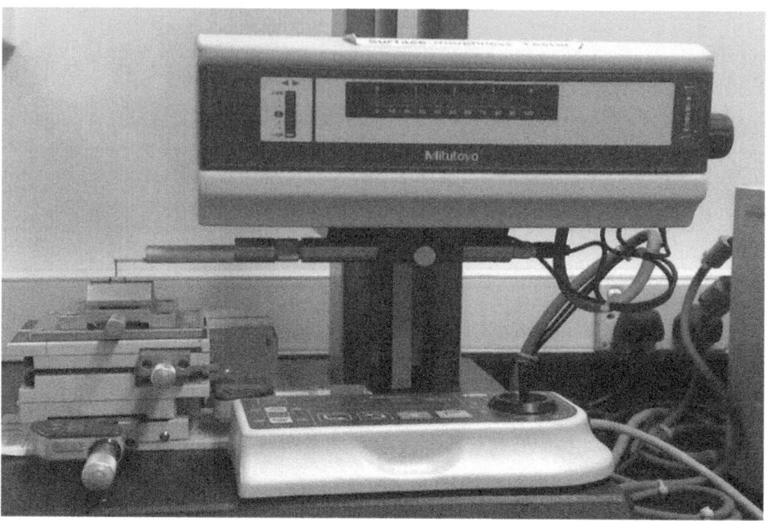

FIGURE 1.4 Surface roughness tester Mitutoyo SV3000.

the least machining cycle time to increase productivity. MRR in grams per minute is the difference of the mass in grams of the workpiece before and after machining to the machining time in minutes. Equation (1.3) was used to determine MRR.

$$MRR = \frac{Mass\,loss\,of\,workpiece}{machining\,\,time} \tag{1.3}$$

The mass loss is measured by weighing the workpiece before and after machining using the electronic balance machine presented in Figure 1.5. The electronic balance machine is from branch Mettler Toledo ME3002. The maximum weight that can be measured is 500 g with the resolution of 0.01 g.

1.10.4 ELECTRODE WEAR RATIO (EWR)

Electrode wear can occur during EDM process and thereby, altering the machining accuracy [20]. Electrode wear types can be volumetric, corner, end and/or side wear. Lead time and additional cost is required to fabricate and replace eroded electrodes. Hence, wear of the electrode must be minimized in EDM process to increase machining efficiency [21]. It is important to study electrode wear and other related factors to improve the machining productivity and process stability. In this present study, EWR is defined as a ratio of electrode mass to that of the workpiece which is expressed as percentage in Equation 1.4 [22]. The mass loss of the electrode and workpiece are measured using electronic balance.

$$EWR = \frac{w_{eb} - w_{ea}}{w_b - w_a} \times 100 \tag{1.4}$$

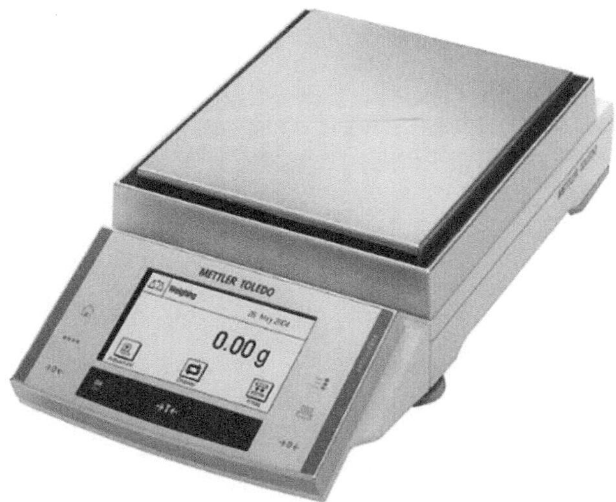

FIGURE 1.5   Electronic precision balance machine.

where:
w_{eb} is the mass of electrode before machining,
w_{ea} is the mass of electrode after machining,
w_b is the mass of workpiece before machining,
w_a is the mass of workpiece after machining,
EWR is the ratio of the electrode mass loss to the material loss in percentage.

1.10.5 Radial Overcut (ROC)

Overcut is the overburn on the workpiece. It is important to determine the ROC to meet high tolerance components requirement to be produced since side wear of electrode can occur. This is necessary for an electrode to be designed properly to meet tolerance requirements. ROC is determined by the half difference of cavity diameter from electrode and workpiece diameter using Equation (1.5) [23].

$$ROC = \frac{D_1 - D_2}{2} \tag{1.5}$$

where: D_1 is the width of electrode and D_2 is the width of workpiece cavity.

According to Ncrisarender et al. [22], the overcut is expressed in Equation (1.5) as half of the difference of diameter of workpiece cavity to the electrode diameter.

1.10.6 Surface Morphology of Machined Surface

EDM is an electro-thermal process which can result in rougher or smooth surface machined surface according to machining parameters setting. Surface roughness

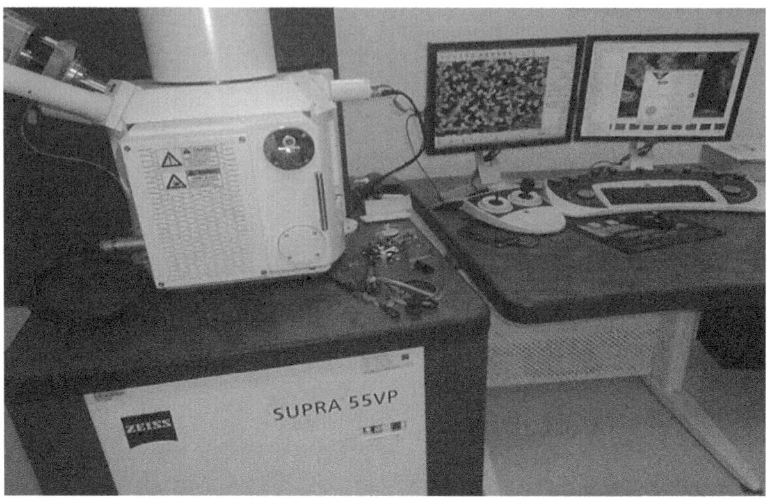

FIGURE 1.6   Field emission scanning electron microscope.

measurement using profile-meter is limited to quantify the surface in term of deviation from its original form. It is important to study the surface morphology of machined surface to conform the result from profile-meter in term of image. From the surface morphology image, defects on machined surface can be characterized in terms of cracks, voids, craters, phase modification which may either be acceptable or rejected depending on application. Specimens were machined using EDM process at various machining parameter settings. Examination of surface morphology of machined surfaces was done on specimens machined at low- and high machining parameters for each category of experiments. FESEM Zeiss SUPRA 55VP presented in Figure 1.6 was used to examine and analyze the machined surfaces. FESEM is a microscope that uses electrons to scan in detail the machined surface as compared to optical microscopy which uses light.

During EDM or PM-EDM process, materials can be transferred from electrode to workpiece and vice versa. The transfer material can be deposited and bound on machined surface improving its hardness and roughness. Therefore, it is important to analyze the materials transferred from electrode or nano aluminum and nano tungsten as evidence of the presence of the transfer elements that contribute to the machined surface enhancement. Analysis of material transfer was done using energy dispersive spectroscopy (EDS) attached to FESEM. EDS analysis involves the generation of an X-ray spectrum from the entire scan area of the SEM.

1.10.7   MICRO-HARDNESS

Hardness testing determines the mechanical property of machined components. Hardness is used to estimate the ductility and resistance to wear, fatigue, and tensile strength properties. Hardness may also be shown to correlate to tensile strength and fatigue in many metals. Measurement of micro-hardness was done using

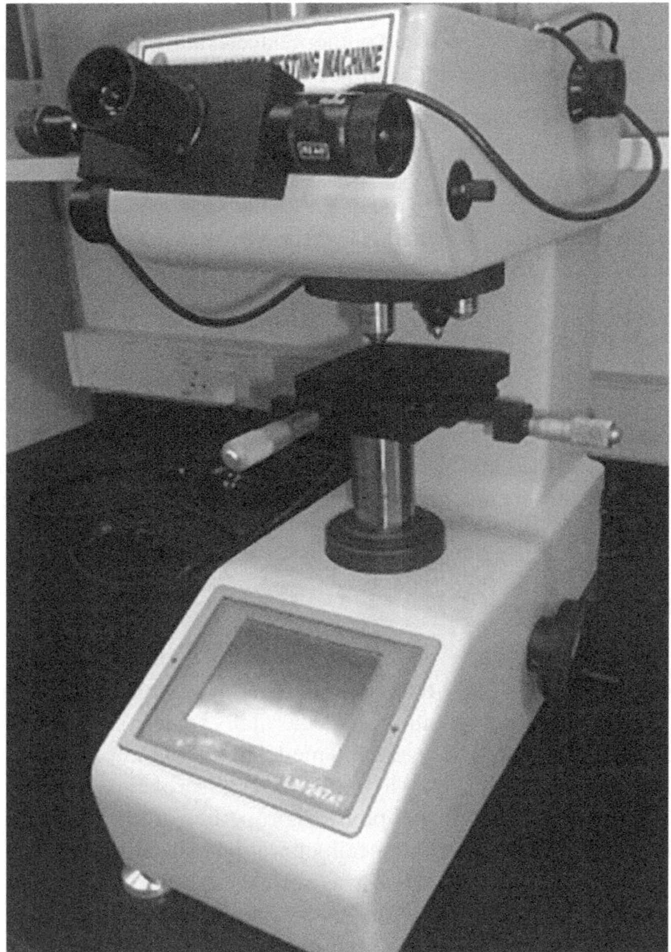

FIGURE 1.7 Image of micro-hardness tester.

micro-hardness tester. ASTM E 384 standard defines and specifies the micro-indentation hardness test method and parameters of materials [24]. Hardness test uses forces in the 1–1000 gf. With the Vickers hardness test, a diamond with top angle of 136° is used. The Vickers hardness parameter is presented in this research project. Tarasov et al. [25] presented in their work, the details of hardness test procedure. Figure 1.7 presents the image of micro-hardness tester.

1.10.8 Fatigue Performance

Fatigue is the progressive and localized structural damage that occurs when a material is subjected to cyclic loading. During EDM or PM-EDM, the repeated electric sparks causes fatigue damage [26]. Fatigue damage includes three stages such as crack initiation, crack propagation, and final fracture. Fatigue of material can also be represented by hardness and some authors have established empirical correlation between hardness and fatigue and ultimate strength in steel as shown in Equations (1.6) and (1.7) [27].

$$\sigma_w = 1.6HV \pm 0.1HV \tag{1.6}$$

where: σ_w is fatigue limit in MPa and HV is the Vickers hardness in kgf/mm² and

$$\sigma_w = 0.5\sigma_u \tag{1.7}$$

where: σ_u is the ultimate tensile strength of material.

In thus study, Equation (1.6) was used to determine the fatigue of the specimen due to specimen shape and steel base material. The shape specimen limits the use of other fatigue testing standards like standard ASTM E606/E606M using rotating cantilever bending fatigue test machine, constant deflection amplitude cantilever bending test machine.

1.10.9 PHASE ANALYSIS

Phase analysis is a quantitative and qualitative non-destructive analysis which is to identify crystalline phases and orientation, to determine structural properties such as strain, grain size, phase composition, and thermal expansion, to determine atomic arrangement. XRD presented in Figure 1.8 model ME510LA2 of Rigaku Corporation Japan available at Universiti Teknologi PETRONAS provides detailed information on the crystallographic structure and physical properties of materials. Due to thermal energy during PM-EDM process, the specimen was heated and melted. Some of melted material was flushed away and some was resolidified and deposited on machined surface. Therefore, phase modifications of machined surface can be examined. The effect of PM-EDM process on phase changes was analyzed using X-ray diffraction (XRD) analysis. XRD provides detailed information on the crystallographic structure and physical properties of materials. XRD measures the average distance between layers or rows of atom and the correspondent intensity. A pattern was obtained in terms of peak position, peak width, and peak intensity which was compared with known standards in the Joint Committee on Powder Diffraction Standards file.

1.10.10 SURFACE SENSITIVITY ANALYSIS

Surface sensitivity analysis provides valuable quantitative and chemical information from the machined surface. Foreign materials from PM-EDM process or from environment can be detected on machined surface. It is important to run surface sensitivity analysis to identify and quantify foreign materials. Surface sensitivity analysis in biomedical engineering is to examine if there is any contamination from foreign elements on machined surface. X-ray photoelectron spectroscopy (XPS) was used to characterize the surface chemical composition of machined surfaces. XPS as

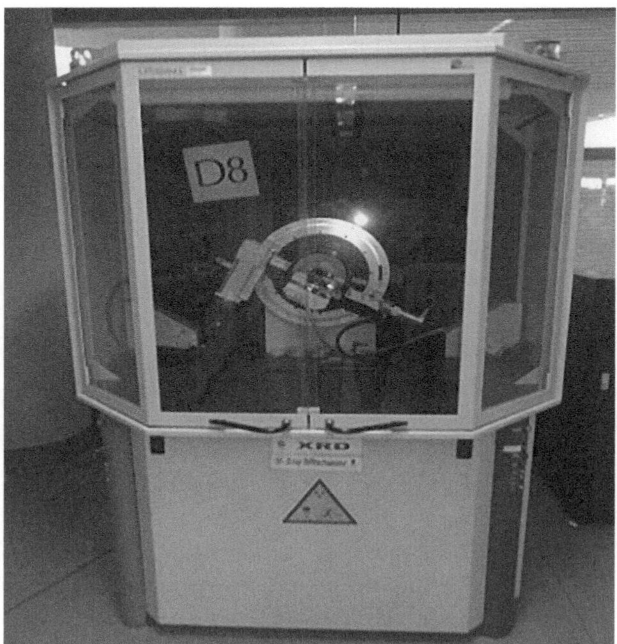

FIGURE 1.8   Powder X-ray diffraction machine.

presented in Figure 1.9 was used to characterize the surface chemical composition of some selected samples. XPS principle is based on the X-ray photon effect that measures the kinetic energy (KE) of collected electrons. The KE of electron depends upon the photon energy (hv) and the binding energy (BE) of electron. By measuring the KE of the emitted electrons, it is possible to determine which elements are near a material's surface, their chemical states, and the BE of electron.

1.10.11   CORROSION TEST

Corrosion analysis is an important parameter indicator for industry and biomedical engineering because corrosion can affect the mechanical properties and biocompatibility of materials. Corrosion analysis was conducted using a linear polarization resistance (LPR) test with three electrodes, according to ASTM G3–89, ASTM G59, and ASTM G31. The use of a three-electrode potentiostat with a separate reference and counter electrode allows the potential and the current at the working electrode (WE) to be measured with little or no "interference" or "contribution" from the other electrodes. Potentiostat polarization measurements were used to study the effect of corrosion on Ti-6Al-4V.

The three electrodes are immersed in a simulated body fluid, Hank's solution as presented in Table 1.7 as the electrolyte. The linear LPR method uses a small voltage of about ±20 mV between the electrodes and the current is measured. The LPR was

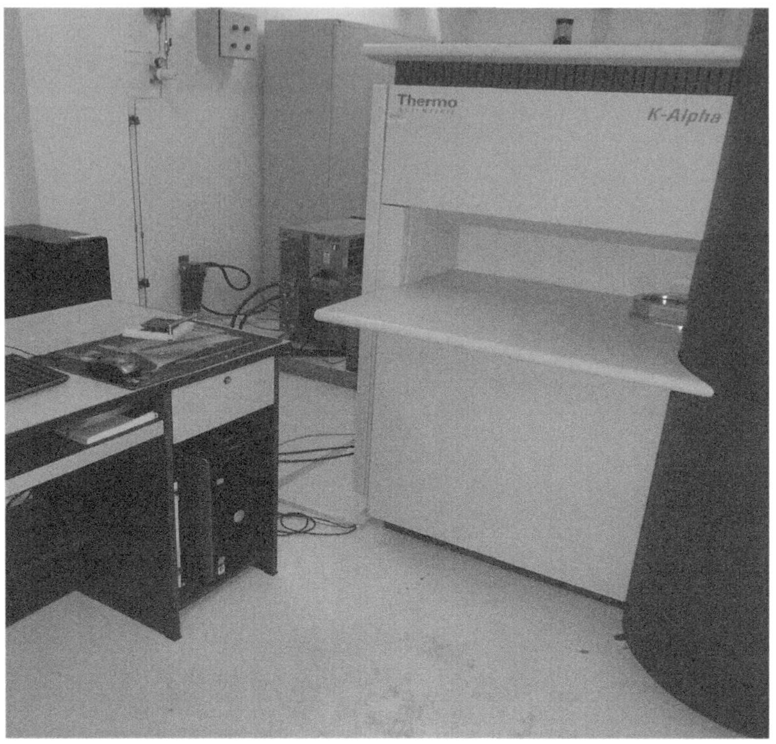

FIGURE 1.9   X-ray photoelectron spectroscopy (XPS).

TABLE 1.7
Hank´s solution chemical composition: simulated body fluid

Component	NaCl	KCl	$CaCl_2$
	Sodium chloride	Potassium chloride	Calcium chloride
(g/L)	8.00	0.40	0.14
Component	$NaHCO_3$	$MgCl_2.6H_2O$	$MgSO_4.7H2O$
	Sodium bicarbonate	Magnesium chloride hexahydrate	Magnesium Sulfate Heptahydrate
(g/L)	0.35	0.60	0.06
Component	Na_2HPO_4	KH_2PO_4	Glucose.2H2O
	Sodium phosphate dibasic	Potassium phosphate monobasic	
(g/L)	0.06	0.60	1.0
Component	pH		
(g/L)	6.8		

done in 3 h setting time with six reading points. Ecor (mV) was ranging from -10 to 10 mV with scan rate of 10 mV/s and sample area of 0.33 cm².

In LPR method, a small current is applied (few µA) therefore, there will be change in electrode potential and current. The potentiostat will measure the potential current changes, plot the overvoltage versus current, and calculate the slope. The measured resistance is inversely related to the corrosion rate.

1.10.12 STATISTICAL ANALYSIS OF OUTPUT RESPONSES

Statistical techniques are used to analyze the output results and the basic techniques are described in this section.

1.11 MATHEMATICAL MODELS

In analysis of an experiment, the models are fitted relating a response to a set of controllable variables. For continuous control variables, the model often fitted can be linear, factorial, or quadratic.

Linear mathematical model (Equation 1.8) is given as follows:

$$Y = \beta_0 + \beta_1 X_1 + \beta_2 X_2 + \beta_i X_i + \varepsilon \tag{1.8}$$

Factorial mathematical model (Equation 1.99):

$$Y = \beta_o + \beta_1 X_1 + \beta_2 X_2 + \beta_{12} X_1 X_2 + \beta_{ij} X_i X_j + \varepsilon \tag{1.9}$$

This allows the effect of changing a control to vary with the setting of another control and $\beta_{ij} X_i X_j$ is the factorial term.

Quadratic mathematical model (Equation 1.10):

$$Y = \beta_o + \beta_1 X_1 + \beta_2 X_2 + \beta_{12} X_1 X_2 + \beta_{11} X_1^2 + \beta_{22} X_2^2 + \beta_{ij} X_i X_j + \beta_{ii} X_i^2 + \varepsilon \tag{1.10}$$

β_i, β_{ii}, β_{ij} represent regression coefficients, β_0 constant coefficient, ε error, X_i and X_j are process variable parameters, and Y is the output response.

1.12 REGRESSION COEFFICIENTS

Regression analysis generates an equation to describe the relationship between machining parameters and output response. Regression coefficients represent the mean change in the response for one unit of change in the parameter while keeping other machining parameters in the model constant. The content of regression coefficients include:

SE Coef.: standard error (SE coef) used for confidence intervals and to perform hypothesis tests.

T-value: the T statistic tests the hypothesis and is the ratio of the sample regression coefficient to its standard error.

P-value: probability that tests the null hypothesis. A p-value <0.05 indicates that the null hypothesis can be rejected. For some parameters, even though p-value is low, it can be meaningful to the model for the interaction effect.

S: standard error (S) of the regression and it is the measure of how well the model fits the data. A smaller value of S is better because it indicates that the data points are closer to the fitted line.

R-Sq: R-squared (R^2) is the squared multiple correlation coefficient or the coefficient of determination.

R-Sq(adj): adjusted R^2 (R-Sq(adj)) is an R^2-like measure after removing the non-significant terms.

1.13 ANALYSIS OF VARIANCE

ANOVA evaluates the null hypothesis that the means for all the groups are the same. In order to test this hypothesis, a Fisher statistic is calculated which compares the variation among the groups. The fitted model plot, interaction plots, and ANOVA are examined. These plots and statistics are needed to determine if the model fit is satisfactory or not. Equation (1.11) is used to determine R^2 which is a statistical measure of how closely the data fit the model.

$$R^2 = \frac{SSB}{SSB + SSE} = \frac{SSB}{SST} \tag{1.11}$$

R^2 is between 0 and 100%. When R-squared is 0%, it indicates that none of the variability of the response data is around its mean. If R-squared is 100%, the model explains that all the variability is around the mean. The higher the R-squared is, the better the model fits the data. Low R-squared values are not always bad and high R^2 values are not always good. Even though R^2 is low, the model terms are statistically significant, conclusions can still be drawn regarding how changes in the parameters affect the output responses. Table 1.8 presents the calculation of mean sources of variance.

Adj SS: adjusted sums of squares (Adj SS) measure the variation for different terms of the model.

Adj MS: adjusted mean squares (Adj MS) measure how much variation a term or a model explains, assuming that all other terms are in the model.

Residual error: estimating the deference between two terms means.

Lack-of-fit: error that occurs when data contain replicates, and it is to determine whether the model accurately fits the data model.

Pure error: pure error occurs for repeated values of dependent variable, Y for a fixed value of independent variable.

TABLE 1.8
Mean sources of variance formula

Source	Sum of squares	df	Mean square	F-ratio	*P*-value
Between groups	SS_B $nS\sum_{i=1}^{k}\left(\bar{y}_i - \bar{\bar{y}}\right)^2$	k - 1	$MS_B = SSB/(k-1)$	$F = MS_B/MS_W$	$F_{k-1,nk-k}$ Chart
Within groups	SS_W $\sum_{i=1}^{k}\sum_{j=i}^{nS}\left(y_{ij} - \bar{y}_i\right)^2$	n - k	$MSW = SS_W/(n-k)$		
Total (Corr.)	SS_T $SST = \sum_{i=1}^{k}\sum_{j=1}^{n_s}\left(y_{ij} - \bar{\bar{y}}\right)^2$	n - 1	$MS_B + MS_W$		

k is number of treatments; n is number of observations.

1.14 STATISTICAL ANALYSIS OPTIONS

Some statistical analysis including diagnostic plots of residual, normal probability plots, contour, and 3D plots are used to evaluate and analysis the model and descripted as follow. Various model graphs can be plotted to show how the output response varies with changes in machining parameters. Model graphs can include one factor plot to show effect of one factor only while other parameters are kept constant; interaction plot which shows how the effect of changing one parameter varies with changes in a second parameter; contour plot which shows the 2D effect and 3D surface.

Interaction graph: plot presenting how the effect of changing one parameter varies with changes in a second parameter.

Contour plot: plot showing the effect of two machining parameters on output response.

3D graph: shows the effects of three machining parameters on output response as shown in Figure 1.10.

Main-effects chart: the chart of average responses versus the factor levels is called the main-effects chart. Plots of main-effect charts in experimental data analysis are the same as in classical experimental data analysis.

1.15 OPTIMIZATION

The objective of optimization in any analysis of a response surface is to find variable parameters levels that produce an optimum output response, or at least a response that is acceptable. Experimental strategies to locate the optimum on a response surface include modeling methods in which a suitable mathematical model of the response surface is built.

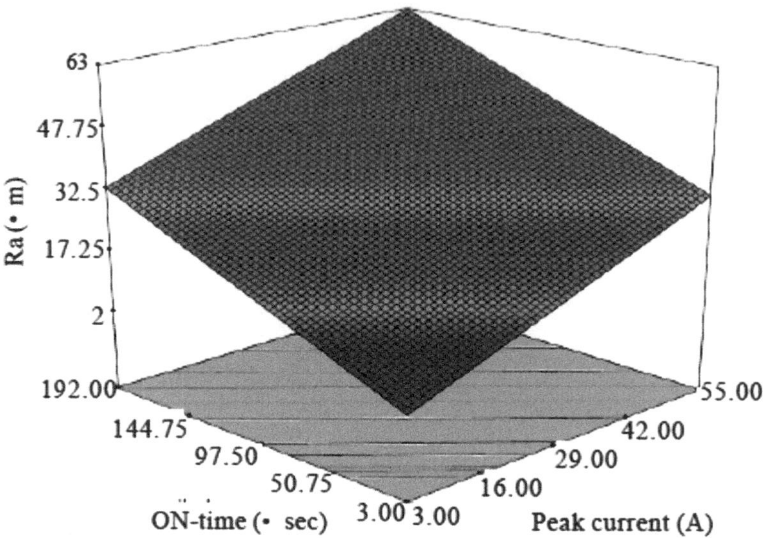

FIGURE 1.10   Corrosion cell.

1.16   CONFIRMATION TEST

The purpose of the confirmation experiment is to attest the validity of the outcomes obtained during the analysis phase. The predicted and actual values from confirmation runs were compared by calculating the error (Equation 1.12).

$$\text{Error}\,(\%) = \frac{\text{Actual value} - \text{Pr\,edicted value}}{\text{Actual value}} \tag{1.12}$$

1.17   RESULTS AND DISCUSSION

1.17.1   REGRESSION COEFFICIENTS FOR RA OF EDM ON TITANIUM ALLOY

Table 1.9 presents the estimated regression coefficients; it can be observed that IP and interaction of ON and interaction ON*GapV having p-value less than 0.05 are the most important parameters. The mathematical model surface roughness of EDM on titanium alloy and the considered process variables was obtained within 95% confidence interval after reducing the not significant terms as follows (Equation 1.13):

$$\text{Ra} = + 9.41 + 1.78^*A + 0.54^*B - 0.54^*C - 1.23^*B^*C \tag{1.13}$$

where: A is peak current IP; B, ON, and C, Gap voltage.

TABLE 1.9
Regression coefficients for Ra of EDM on titanium alloy

Term	Coef	SE Coef	T	P
Constant	10.2832	0.6222	16.527	0.000
IP	1.7652	0.4678	3.773	0.001
ON	0.5427	0.4678	1.160	0.260
GapV	-0.4962	0.4678	-1.061	0.301
IP*IP	-1.3898	1.1868	-1.171	0.255
ON*ON	0.3156	1.1779	0.268	0.791
GapV*GapV	-0.2671	1.2043	-0.222	0.827
IP*ON	0.0079	0.4959	0.016	0.987
IP*GapV	-0.8121	0.4954	-1.639	0.117
ON*GapV	-1.2333	0.4956	-2.489	0.022

$S = 1.985$ R-Sq = 59.0% R-Sq(adj) = 40.5%

TABLE 1.10
ANOVA for Ra of EDM on titanium alloy

Source	df	Seq SS	Adj SS	Adj MS	F	P
Regression	9	113.30	113.30	12.589	3.20	0.015
Linear	3	65.26	65.81	21.936	5.57	0.006
Square	3	13.07	13.19	4.398	1.12	0.366
Interaction	3	34.98	34.98	11.659	2.96	0.057
Residual error	20	78.77	78.77	3.938		
Lack-of-fit	5	43.40	43.40	8.679	3.68	0.023
Pure error	15	35.37	35.37	2.358		
Total	29	192.07				

1.17.2 ANALYSIS OF VARIANCE FOR RA OF EDM ON TITANIUM ALLOY

Table 1.10 presents the ANOVA for Ra when machining titanium alloy EDM and surfactant. With regression p-value of 0.015, the results fit the model with lack-of-fit of 3.68.

F ratios are calculated for 95% level of confidence and the factors having p-value more than 0.05 are considered non-significant. The model adequacy checking includes the test for significance of the regression model, model coefficients, and lack-of-fit, which is carried out subsequently using ANOVA on the curtailed model. The total error on regression is the sum of errors on linear, square, and interactions terms (113.30 = 65.26 + 13.07 + 34.98). The residual error is the sum of pure and lack-of-fit errors (78.77 = 43.40 + 35.37). The fit summary recommended that the linear model is statistically significant for analysis of surface roughness with linear F of 21.06. In Table 10, p-value for the lack-of-fit is 3.68, which is not significant, so the model is adequate. Moreover, the mean square error of pure error is less than that of lack-of-fit.

1.17.3 Effects Plot for Ra of EDM on Titanium Alloy

Figure 1.11 presents the main effect of IP, ON-time, and gap voltage on Ra. Ra is getting rougher when IP and ON-time vary from low to high setting value. Ra slightly increases with variation of gap voltage from 80 to 110 V, but it remains slightly constant around Ra value of 10 µm from 110 to 150 V. This can be due to high thermal conductivity dissipate heat rapidly through the workpiece resulting in a low value of Ra. Kiyak and Çakır [14] stated similar effect in their finding that higher peak current resulted in higher surface roughness due to higher thermal loading into the workpiece and electrode.

1.17.4 Interaction Plot for Ra of EDM on Titanium Alloy

Figure 1.12 shows the interaction effects of machining parameters and the change in level of one or two machining parameters affect the output response. There is interaction between any two machining parameters combinations.

Figure 1.13 presents a 3D surface response for Ra subjected to the machining parameters of IP and ON-time, while gap voltage remains constant at the center point

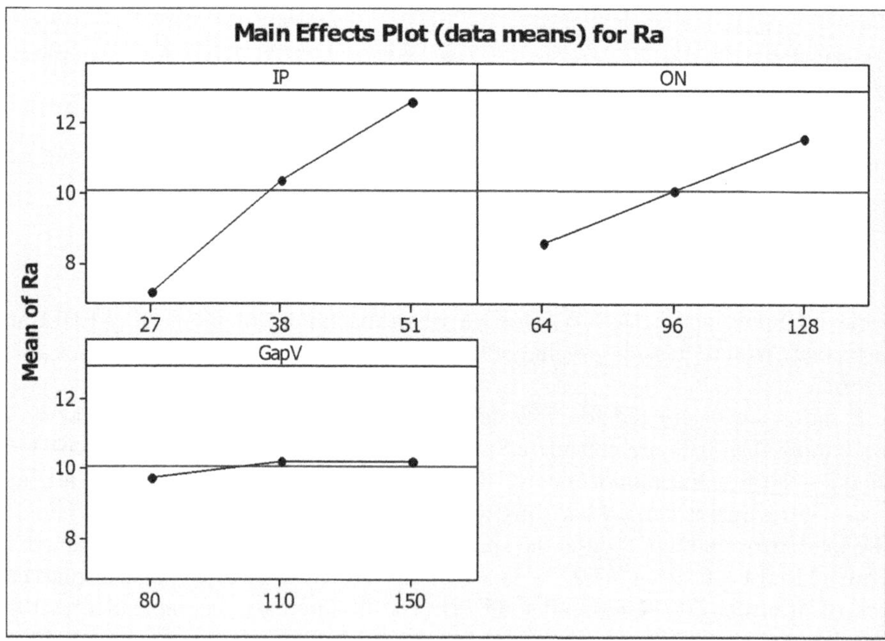

FIGURE 1.11 Effects plot for Ra (µm) of EDM on titanium alloy.

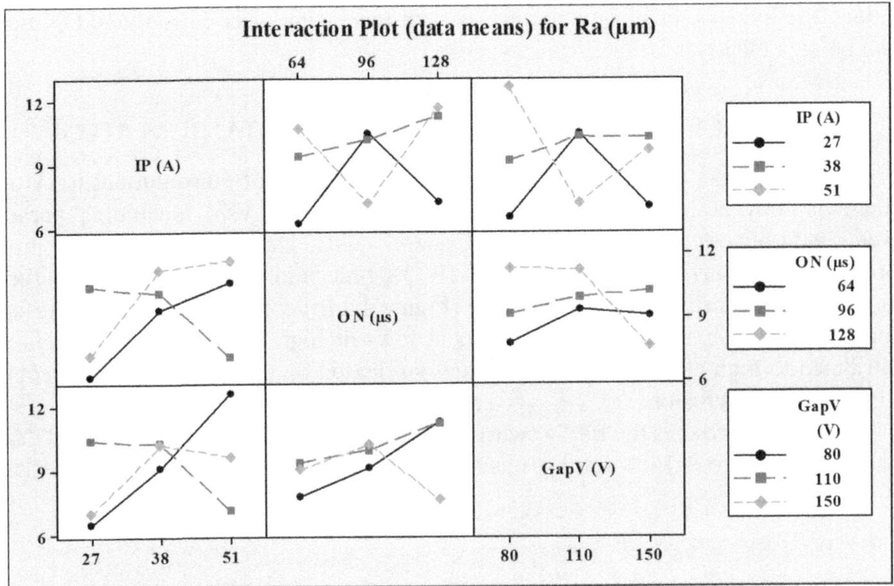

FIGURE 1.12 Interaction plot for Ra of EDM on titanium alloy.

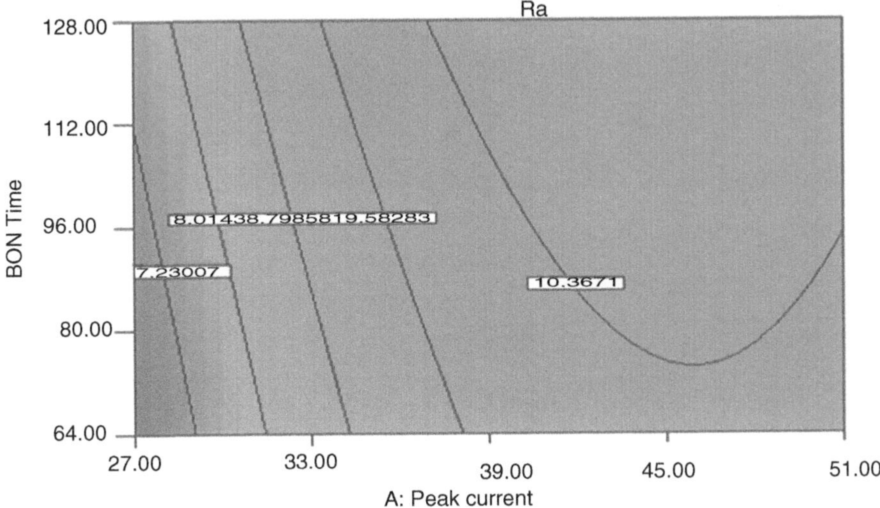

FIGURE 1.13 Contour plot for Ra of EDM on titanium alloy.

value. The increase in surface roughness with increasing peak current and ON-time can be seen clearly.

1.18 SURFACE MORPHOLOGY OF EDM ON TITANIUM ALLOY

Figure 1.14 shows the morphology of machined surface of conventional EDM on titanium alloy at low (Figure1.14a) and high (Figure 1.19b) machining parameter conditions as mentioned above. Craters, voids, and micro-cracks are more pronounced on surface machined at high IP, ON-time, and gap voltage. Non-uniform agglomerates distribution on the surface (Figure 1.14b) contributes to higher surface roughness. Conventional EDM, whether at low- or high machining parameters, is attributed to high electrical discharge energy released on the surface during electro-discharge spark erosion.

Figure 1.15 presents the EDS spectrum of machined surfaces at low (Figure 1.15a) and high (Figure 1.15b) setting machining parameters. As mentioned for EDM

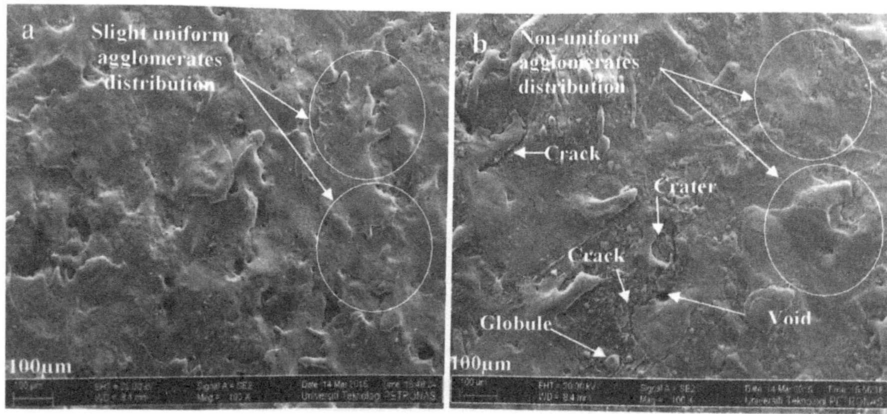

FIGURE 1.14 EDM surface morphology.

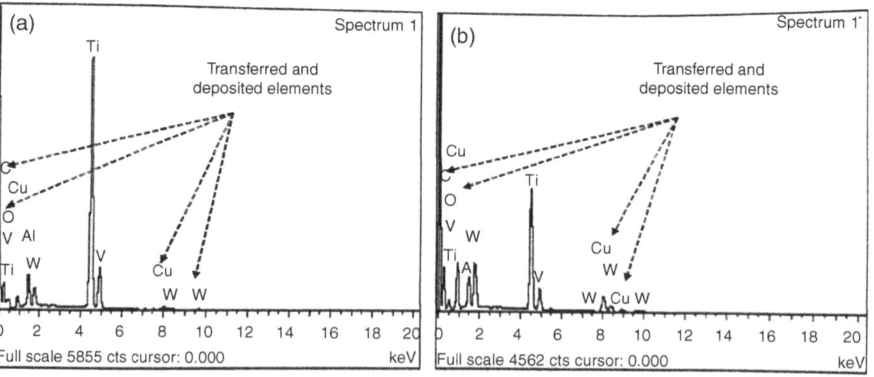

FIGURE 1.15 a and b EDS EDM on titanium alloy at low machining parameters.

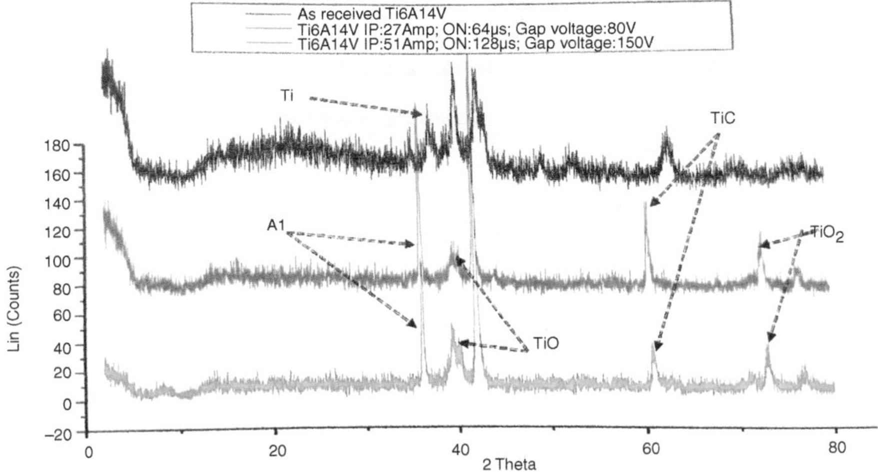

FIGURE 1.16   XRD on titanium alloy machined surface.

machined surfaces, materials were transferred from the electrode to the workpiece during EDM. The presence of copper, tungsten, carbon, and oxygen is observed. The amount of carbon, copper, and tungsten are more pronounced at high parameters setting. These alloying elements deposited and embedded on machined surface not only reduce the cracks, craters, and voids but also improve the machined surface properties particularly the corrosion resistance.

1.19   PHASE ANALYSIS OF EDM ON TITANIUM ALLOY

Figure 1.16 presents the XRD pattern on titanium alloy machined using EDM. The highest peaks occurred at 2 theta value of around 42.174 (Cu Ka) and it can be observed the presence of TiC, Ti, and TiO_2 phases on the machined surface.

1.20   MATERIAL REMOVAL RATE OF EDM ON TITANIUM ALLOY

MRR of conventional EDM on titanium alloy was determined and presented in this section.

1.20.1   EFFECTS PLOT FOR MRR OF EDM ON TITANIUM ALLOY

Figure 1.17 presents the effects of IP, ON-time, and gap voltage on MRR. MRR is increasing with the variation of IP and ON-time from low- to center point values and it decreases from the center point to high values. During the EDM process, the effect IP is proportional to MRR from 27 to 38 A after which MRR trend remains slightly constant from 38 to 51 A. The increase in MRR when IP varies from low- to high set values is due to the produced intense discharge spark rising in temperature,

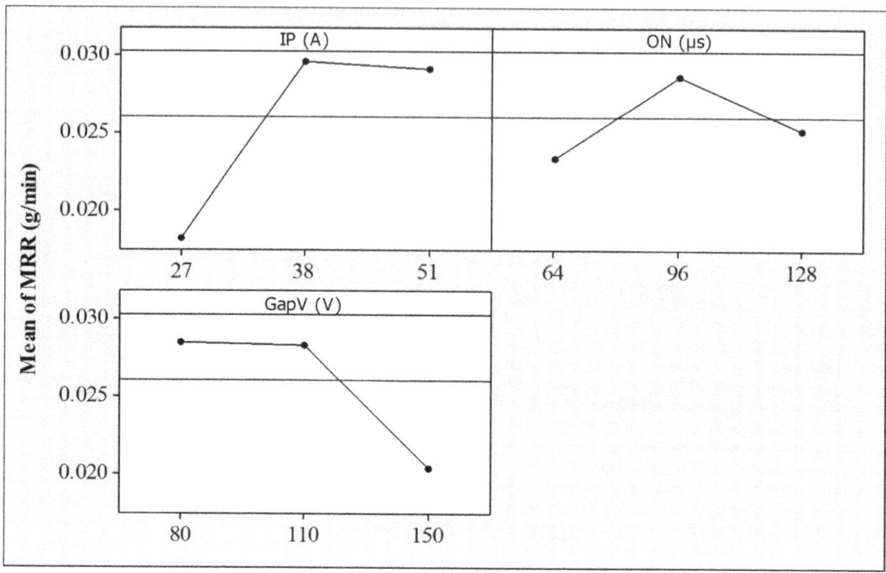

FIGURE 1.17   Effects plot for MRR of EDM on titanium alloy.

which heats the machining area causing more material to melt and erode from the workpiece.

1.20.2 Interaction Plot for MRR of EDM on Titanium Alloy

Figure 1.18 shows the interaction between three different machining parameters, especially IP, ON-time, and gap voltage on MRR. This explains that the effect of one factor is dependent upon another factor. The spark energy increases with IP, ON-time hence, more MRR is achieved with IP, ON-time. The decrease in MRR is because with higher ON-time and gap voltage, the sparks formed between the electrode and workpiece obstruct the energy transfer and thus reduces MRR.

1.21 ELECTRODE WEAR RATIO OF EDM ON TITANIUM ALLOY

1.21.1 Plot for EWR of EDM on Titanium Alloy

Figure 1.19 presents the main effect of IP, ON-time, and gap voltage on EWR when machining titanium alloy using conventional EDM. EWR is getting wider and more pronounced when varying IP and ON-time voltage from the low- to high-setting value. EWR is slightly low with ON-time varying from low- to high-setting value. During the conventional EDM process on titanium alloy Ti-6Al-4V, machining parameters especially IP, ON-time, and gap voltage impact on the EWR as shown in main effect plot of EWR. As the IP, ON-time, and gap voltage vary from low to the high set of values, the EWR is increased. This happened because IP, ON-time, and gap voltage contribute to increase the discharge energy, and thus more heat energy is generated on

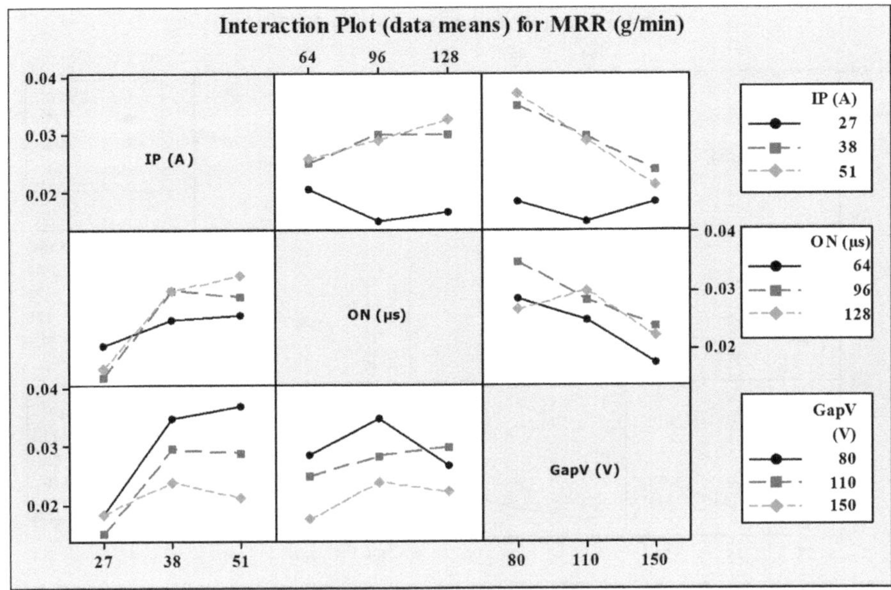

FIGURE 1.18 Interaction plot for MRR of EDM on MHSS.

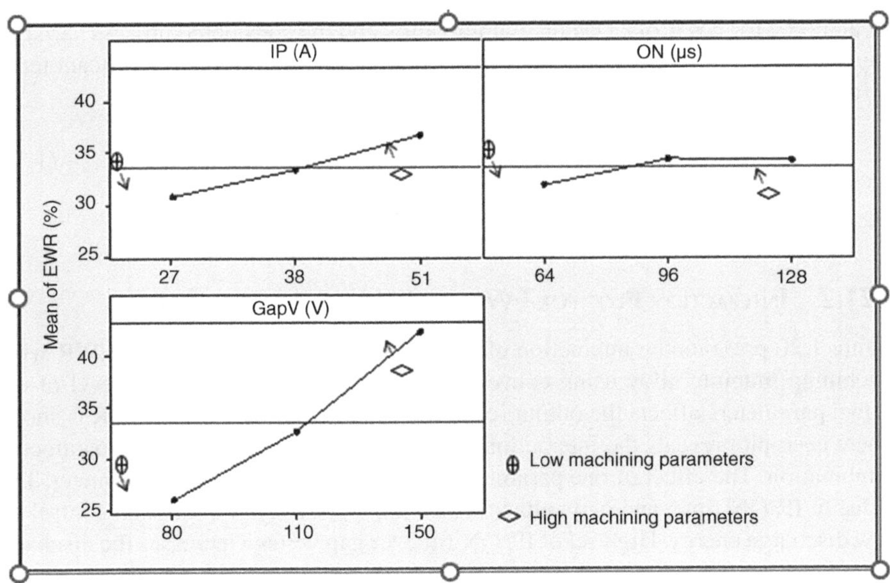

FIGURE 1.19 Effects plot for EWR of EDM on titanium alloy.

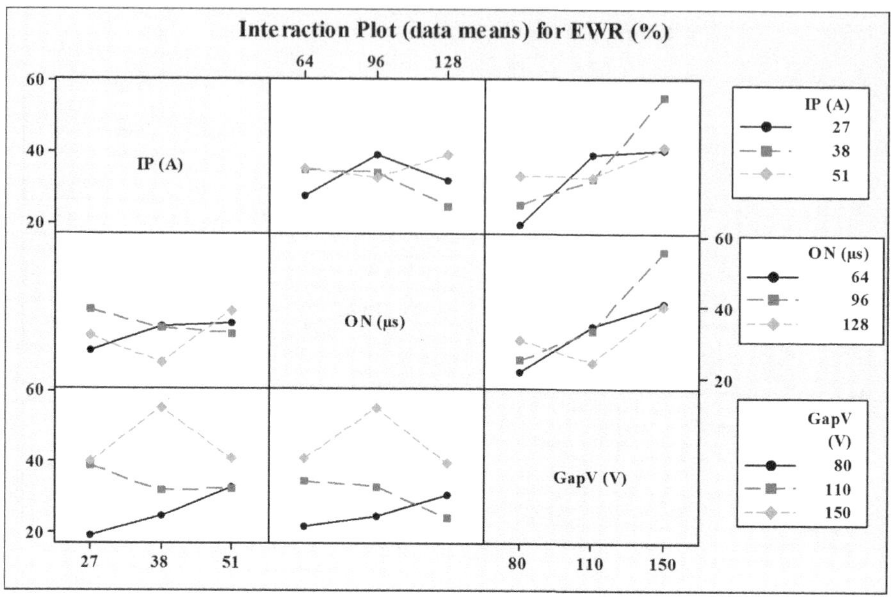

FIGURE 1.20 Interaction plot for EWR of EDM on titanium alloy.

the electrode area leading to more material removed from the electrode. The mathematical model for EWR of EDM on titanium alloy and the considered process variables was obtained within 95% confidence interval after reducing the not significant terms as follows (Equation 1.14):

$$EWR = +34.34 +3.43*A +7.64*C -3.74*A*C \qquad (1.14)$$

where: A is peak current IP and C, Gap voltage.

1.21.2 Interaction Plot for EWR of EDM on Titanium Alloy

Figure 1.20 presents the interaction effects of machining parameters on EWR when machining titanium alloy using conventional EDM. The change in the level of one or two parameters affects the output response. The interaction plot of EWR is shown where each plot reveals the interaction between two different machining parameters combination. The effect of one parameter is dependent upon another parameter. This is due to IP, ON-time, and gap voltage which independently or combined control the flow discharge energy. High set of IP, ON-time, or gap voltage increases the discharge energy.

1.22 RADIAL OVERCUT OF EDM ON TITANIUM ALLOY

The radical overcut of conventional EDM on titanium alloy use was determined and presented in this section.

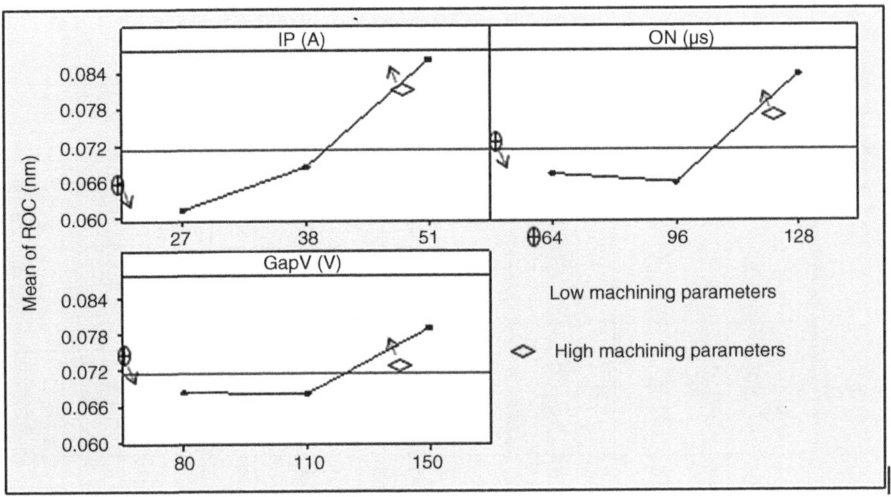

FIGURE 1.21   Effects plot for ROC of EDM on titanium alloy.

1.22.1 Effects Plot for ROC of EDM on Titanium Alloy

Figure 1.21 presents the effect plot of IP, ON-time, and gap voltage on ROC when machining titanium alloy using conventional EDM. ROC is getting larger with the increase of IP, ON-time, and gap voltage. The increase in discharge energy induces more removal material from the lateral side of electrode. The regression coefficients for ROC with $R^2 = 55.5\%$ indicate that the model can predict the response with high accuracy. The standard deviation of errors in ROC the model is S = 0.01894 indicates that the observed data are closer to the fitted line. The mathematical model for ROC of EDM on titanium alloy and the considered process variables was obtained within 95% confidence interval after reducing the not significant terms as shown in equation (1.15).

$$ROC = +0.063 +0.011*A +8.333E\text{-}003*B +0.012*B^\wedge 2 \tag{1.15}$$

where: A is peak current IP and B, ON-time.

1.22.2 Interaction Plot for ROC of EDM on Titanium Alloy

Figure 1.22 shows the interaction effects of machining parameters when machining titanium alloy using conventional EDM and the change in the level of one or two parameters affects the output response. ROC increases with the increase of ON-time and gap voltage. The interaction plot of ROC shows the interaction between the three different machining parameters such as IP, ON-time, and gap voltage.

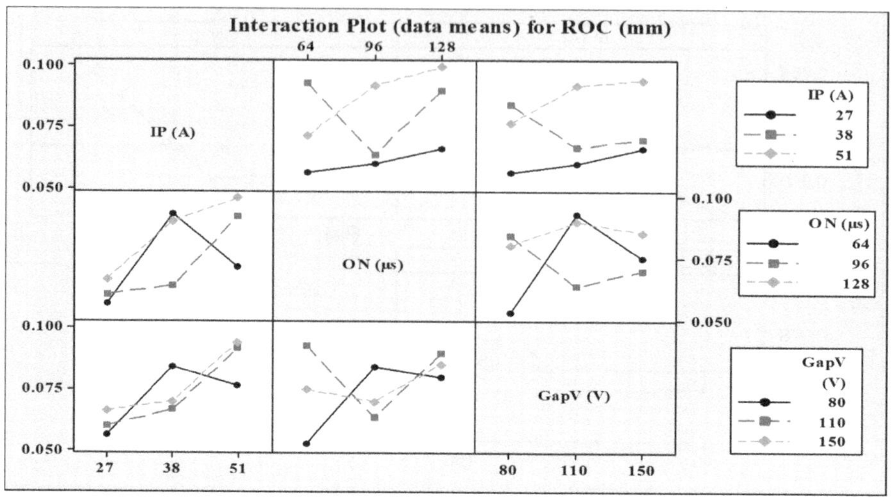

FIGURE 1.22   Interaction plot for ROC of EDM on titanium alloy.

1.23 SURFACE ROUGHNESS OF EDM ON MOLYBDENUM HIGH-SPEED STEEL

Average surface roughness (Ra) of conventional EDM on molybdenum high-speed steel was determined and presented in this section.

1.23.1 REGRESSION COEFFICIENTS FOR RA OF EDM ON MHSS

Table 1.11 presents the estimated regression coefficients. Regression coefficients represent the mean change in the response for one unit of change in the parameter while keeping other machining parameters in the model constant. From Table 1.11, it indicates that peak current and ON-time have significant effect on output response followed by ON-time. The mathematical model for correlating the surface roughness of EDM on molybdenum workpiece material and the considered process variables was obtained within 95% confidence interval after reducing the not significant terms as follows (Equation 1.16):

$$Ra = +12.25 +2.25 *A +0.84*B -0.61*A*B \tag{1.16}$$

where: A is peak current IP and B, ON-time.

1.23.2 ANALYSIS OF VARIANCE (ANOVA) FOR RA OF EDM ON MHSS

Table 1.12 presents the ANOVA of Ra. The *p*-value 0.000 indicates that the model is well fitted. The total error on regression is the sum of errors on linear, square, and interactions terms (125.325 = 117.235 + 3.494 + 4.596).

TABLE 1.11
Regression coefficient for Ra of EDM on MHSS

Term	Coef	SE Coef	T	P
Constant	12.6802	0.4283	29.607	0.000
IP	2.3657	0.3220	7.346	0.000
ON	0.8946	0.3220	2.778	0.012
GapV	0.3685	0.3220	1.145	0.266
IP*IP	0.0395	0.8169	0.048	0.962
ON*ON	0.6926	0.8108	0.854	0.403
GapV*GapV	-1.0987	0.8290	-1.325	0.200
IP*ON	-0.4784	0.3414	-1.401	0.176
IP*GapV	0.0698	0.3410	0.205	0.840
ON*GapV	0.2218	0.3411	0.650	0.523

S = 1.366 R-Sq = 77.0% R-Sq(adj) = 66.7%

TABLE 1.12
ANOVA for Ra of EDM on MHSS

Source	DF	Seq SS	Adj SS	Adj MS	F	P
Regression	9	125.257	125.257	13.9174	7.46	0.000
Linear	3	116.847	117.547	39.1823	21.00	0.000
Square	3	3.882	3.877	1.2925	0.69	0.567
Interaction	3	4.527	4.527	1.5091	0.81	0.504
Residual error	20	37.320	37.320	1.8660		
Lack-of-fit	5	3.489	3.489	0.6978	0.31	0.900
Pure error	15	33.832	33.832	2.2554		
Total	29	162.577				

The residual error is the total of pure and lack-of-fit errors (37.252 = 33.832+ 3.421). In Table 12, the lack-of-fit p-value is 0.90, which is not significant, so the model is adequate. The mean square error of pure error is less than that of lack-of-fit.

1.23.3 Effects Plot for Ra of EDM on MHSS

The effects of EDM machining parameters on the surface roughness of molybdenum high-speed steel are recorded and presented in Figure 1.23. The influence of the peak current supplied to the electrode on Ra was analyzed by keeping the ON-time and gap voltage. As the current is increased from 27 to 51 A, the Ra machined surface increases as it can be seen with regression squared (R^2) =0. 771. As the peak current is increased to 51 A, the Ra of the machined surface is about 16 µm. Higher IP caused a poorer surface finish of molybdenum high-speed steel. The peak current determines the size of spark energy. By increasing the peak current, the spark energy increases which creates more craters and cracks leading to increasing surface roughness.

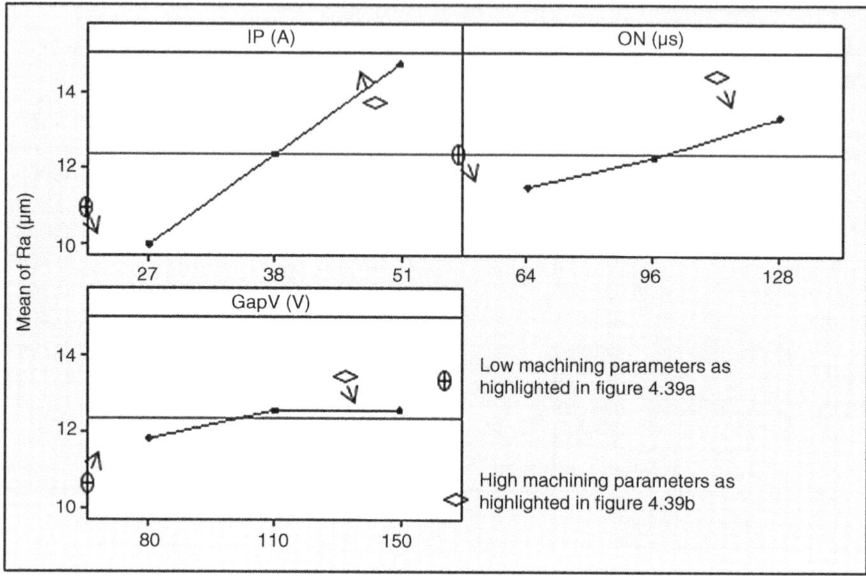

FIGURE 1.23   Effects plot for Ra of EDM on MHSS.

Narender et al. found that higher peak current resulted in higher surface roughness due to higher thermal loading into the workpiece and electrode [22].

1.23.4   INTERACTION PLOT FOR RA OF EDM ON MHSS

Figure 1.24 presents the interaction effects of EDM machining parameters on surface roughness (Ra). An interaction effect of parameters on Ra occurs when the effect of one parameter changes depending on the level of another parameter as it can be analyzed, there is an interaction effect of machining parameters on the Ra. This is because the three machining parameters IP, ON-time, and gap voltage determine the size of discharge energy.

1.24   SURFACE MORPHOLOGY OF EDM ON MHSS

EDM process creates alterations layer on the machined surface. The alterations on the machined surface vary according to the machining parameters setting. These damages layers are formed in relation to the surface roughness of the workpiece. The depth and characteristics of surface morphology are studied using FESEM for some selected parameter settings. Figure 1.25 presents the surface morphology of machined surfaces as the result of changes in IP, ON-time, and gap voltage at low- and high parameter setting. Machined surface micrograph at low IP, ON-time, and gap voltage shows a less rough surface. Craters, voids, and micro-cracks can be analyzed especially for samples machined at high IP, ON-time, and gap voltage. It can be analyzed that the

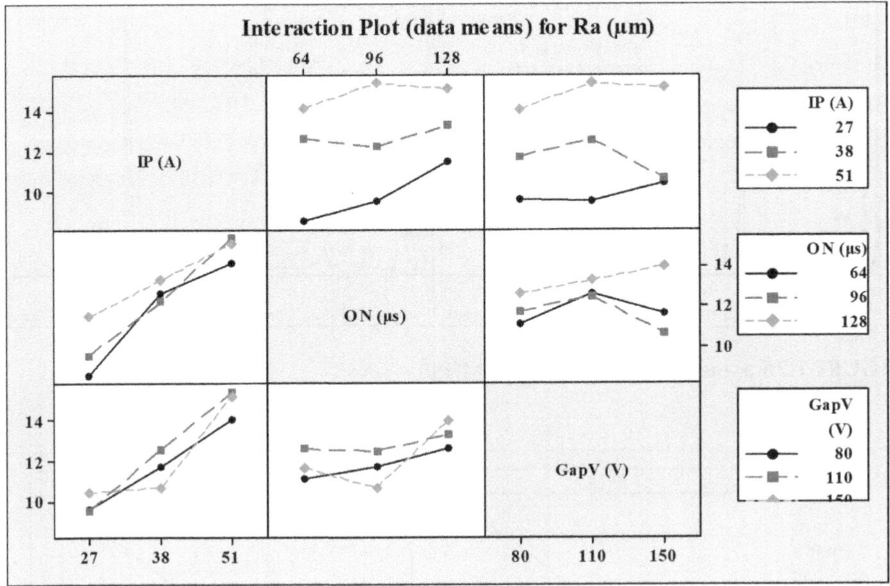

FIGURE 1.24   Interaction plot for Ra of EDM on MHSS.

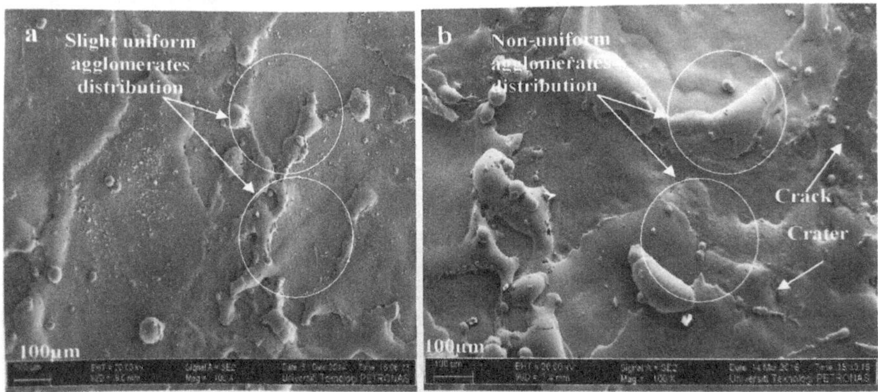

FIGURE 1.25   EDM surface morphology.

surface becomes rougher with an increase in IP, ON-time, and gap voltage. With the increase of IP, ON-time, and gap voltage, electrical discharge energy increases which induces rougher on the machined surface.

Figure 1.26a and b presents EDS spectrum of EDM on molybdenum high-speed steel at low- and high machining parameters setting. The presence of carbon, oxygen, and copper is detected on machined surface with increase in number of alloying elements as compared to as received molybdenum high-speed steel.

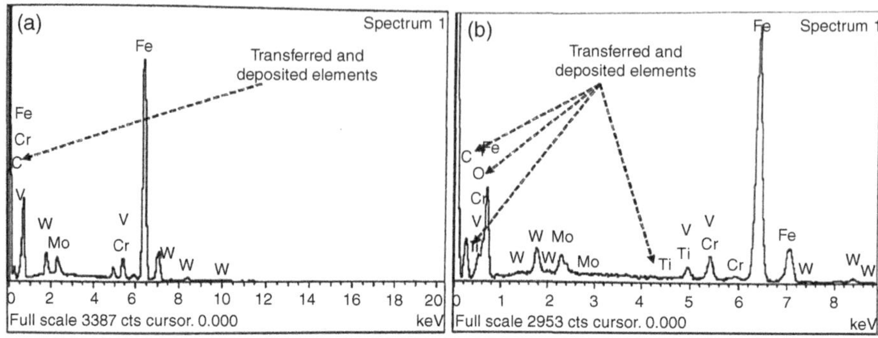

FIGURE 1.26 a and b　EDS of EDM on MHSS.

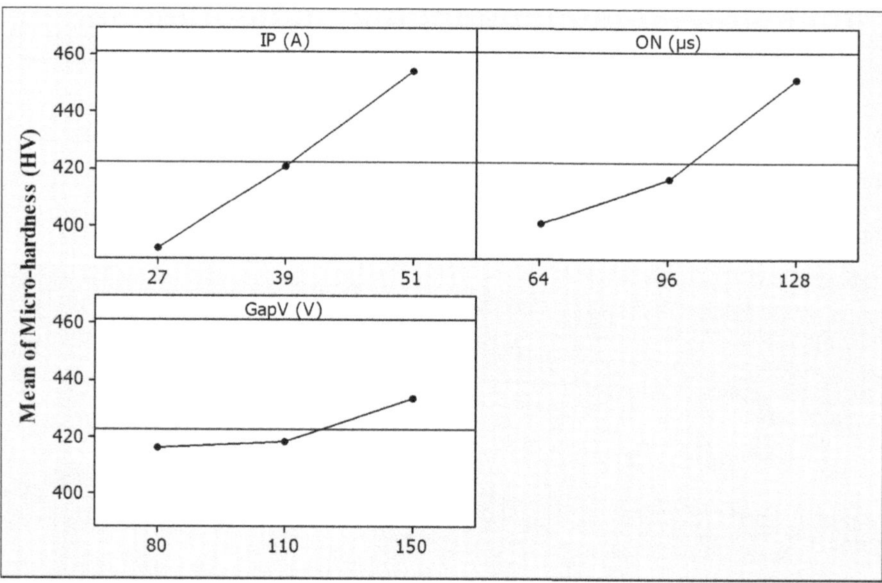

FIGURE 1.27　Micro-hardness of EDM on MHSS.

1.25　MICRO-HARDNESS OF EDM ON MHSS

Figure 1.27 shows the trend of micro-hardness of molybdenum high-speed steel after EDM process and measured using micro-hardness tester on three different locations on the machined surface. The micro-hardness of as received molybdenum high-speed steel is 316.7 HV. The micro-hardness of molybdenum high-speed steel after EDM is higher than the micro-hardness of bulk material as. Micro-hardness of molybdenum high-speed steel after EDM can reach 458 HV which is increased about 44.9% from as received molybdenum high-speed steel micro-hardness.

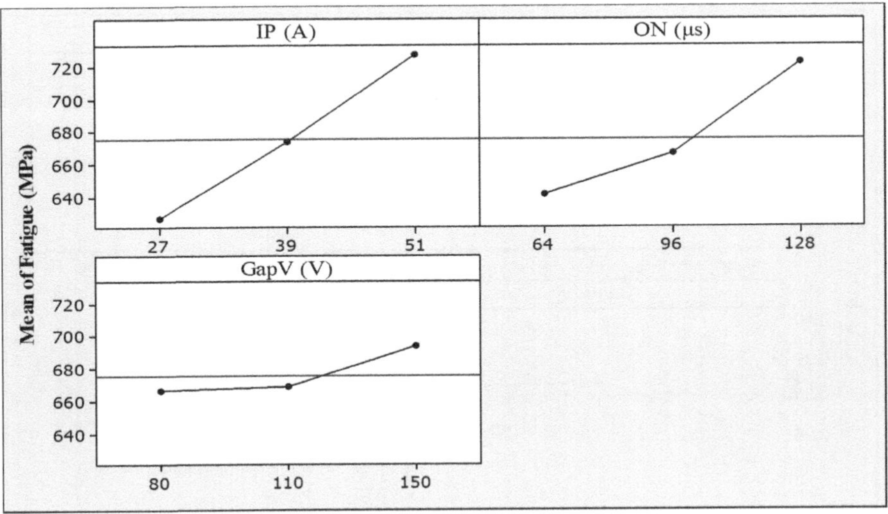

FIGURE 1.28 Fatigue of EDM on MHSS.

1.26 FATIGUE PERFORMANCE OF EDM ON MHSS

Figure 1.28 shows the effect of EDM machining parameters on fatigue performance after EDM process. Fatigue performance of as received molybdenum high-speed steel is about 505.60 MPa. Using $\sigma_w = 1.6HV \pm 0.1HV$, a correlation between hardness in HV and fatigue in MPa stated earlier, it can be found that there is a significant improvement on fatigue performance as compared to the fatigue of bulk molybdenum high-speed material. Improvement of fatigue is due to the handing of the machined surface during EDM process.

1.27 MATERIAL REMOVAL RATE OF EDM ON MOLYBDENUM HIGH-SPEED STEEL

The MRR of conventional EDM on molybdenum high-speed steel was determined and presented in this section.

1.27.1 EFFECTS PLOT FOR MRR OF EDM ON MHSS

Figure 1.29 presents the plot of MRR when machining molybdenum high-speed steel using conventional EDM. IP, ON-time, and gap voltage influence the MRR. The increase in MRR when IP, ON-time, and gap voltage vary from low- to high set values is expected because an increase in peak current, ON-time, and gap voltage produces intense spark, which rose in temperature heating the zone between electrode and workpiece causing more material to be melted and removed from the workpiece. The regression coefficients for MRR are shown. $R^2 = 58.3\%$ indicates that the model can be able to predict the output responses with accuracy. The standard deviation of

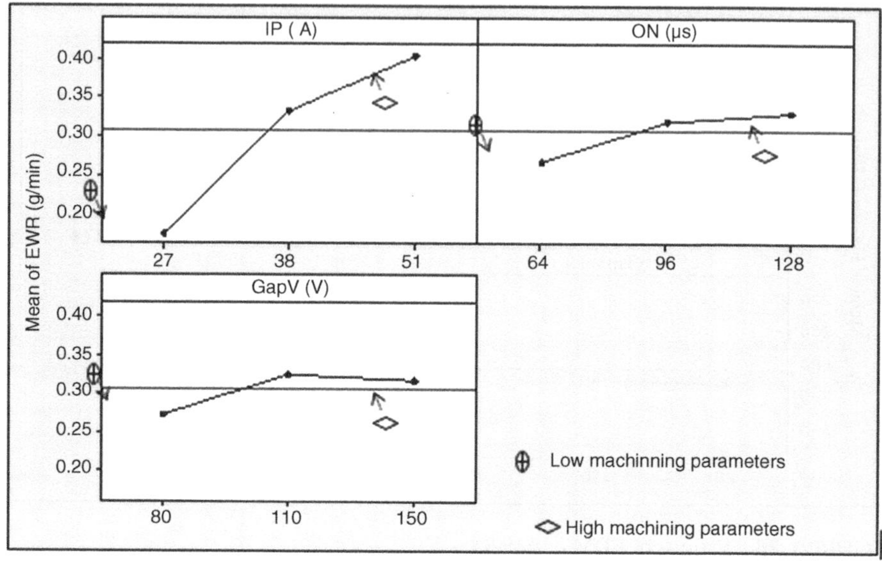

FIGURE 1.29   Effects plot for MRR of EDM on MHSS.

errors in the MRR model is $S = 0.1058$ and this indicates that the observed data are closer to the fitted line.

It indicates that parameters IP and ON-time are significant parameters and interaction effect on MRR of EDM on molybdenum high-speed steel. The mathematical model for MRR of EDM on molybdenum high-speed steel workpiece material and the considered process variables was obtained within 95% confidence interval after reducing the not significant terms as follows:

$$MRR = +0.32 +0.041*A +0.029*B \qquad (1.17)$$

where: A is peak current and B, ON-time.

1.27.2   INTERACTION PLOT FOR MRR OF EDM ON MHSS

Figure 1.30 presents the interaction plot of MRR subjected to machining parameters especially IP, ON-time, and gap voltage. It can be examined that the change in the level of one machining parameter affects the MRR. There is an interaction between any two machining parameters combinations. This explains that the effect of one parameter is dependent upon another parameter, that is why there are no parallel trends in interaction plot. The spark energy increases with IP and ON-time hence, more MRR is achieved with IP, ON-time. The decrease in MRR is because the sparks formed between the electrode and workpiece obstruct the energy transfer and thus reduces MRR.

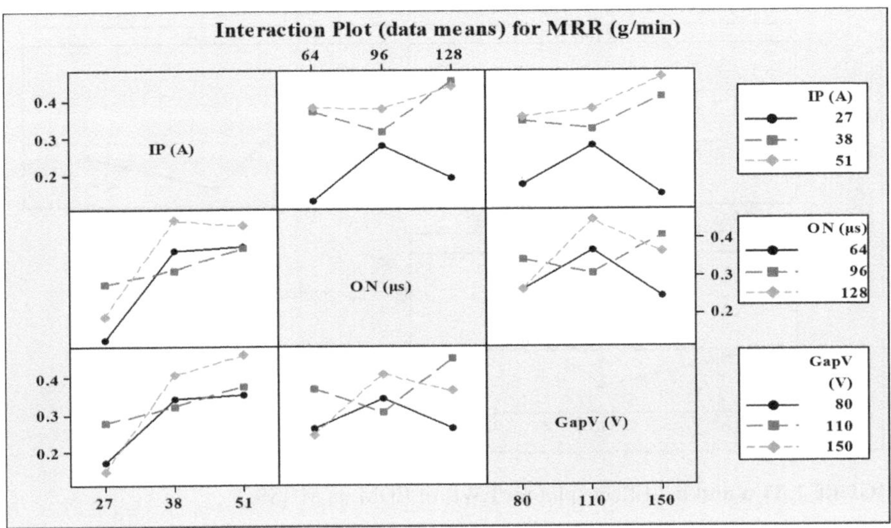

FIGURE 1.30 Interaction plot for MRR of EDM on MHSS.

1.28 ELECTRO WEAR RATIO OF EDM ON MHSS

EWR of conventional EDM on molybdenum high-speed steel was determined and presented in this section.

1.28.1 EFFECTS PLOT FOR EWR OF EDM ON MHSS

Figure 1.31a and b present the main effect of machining parameters on EWR. It analyzed that EWR tends to decrease for low value to the center point of all three parameters. Three machining parameters IP, ON-time, and gap voltage influence on input energy and at the low value of any of three machining parameters, the energy is lower hitting less the electrode, so less wear. When the value of one parameter increases, the discharge also increases and more discharge current hits the electrode removing more material. The regression coefficients for EWR are presented with $R^2 = 61.5\%$ indicate that the model can predict the response with high accuracy. The standard deviation of errors of EWR model which is $S = 0.191$ indicates that the observed data have fallen to the fitted line. It indicates that parameters IP, ON-time, and interaction ON*GapV for EWR of EDM on molybdenum high-speed steel. The mathematical model for EWR of EDM on molybdenum high-speed steel material and the considered process variables was obtained within 95% confidence interval after reducing the not significant terms as follows:

$$EWR = +2.78 +0.33*A -0.54*B +0.34*C -0.71*B*C +1.05*A^2. \quad (1.18)$$

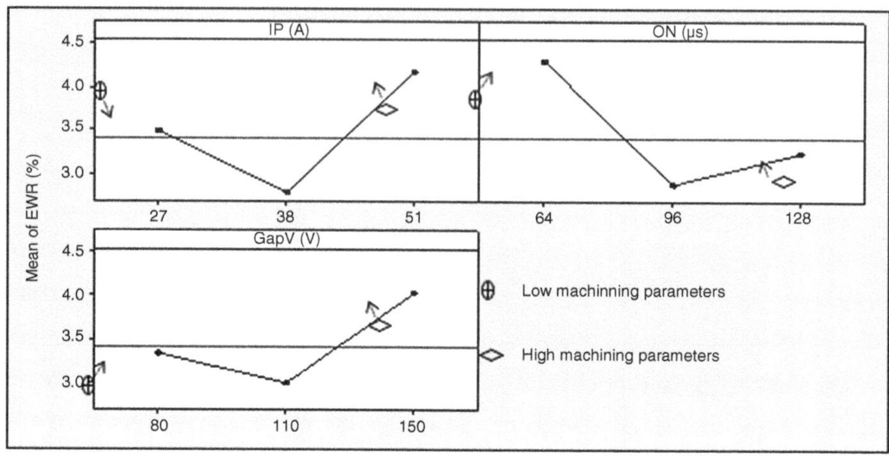

FIGURE 1.31 a and b   Effects plot for EWR of EDM on MHSS.

1.29 RADIAL OVERCUT OF EDM ON MHSS

ROC of electrical discharge machining on molybdenum high-speed steel was determined and presented in this section.

1.29.1 EFFECTS PLOT FOR ROC OF EDM ON MHSS

Figure 1.32 presents the main effect of IP, ON-time, and gap voltage on overcut. Overcut is getting wider when each of the three parameter increases. The increase in discharge energy induces more material removal from the lateral side. The regression coefficients for ROC of EDM on MHSS is $R^2 = 61.2\%$ indicates that the model can predict the output response with accuracy. The standard deviation of errors of the ROC model is $S = 0.01495$ and it indicates that the observed data are closer to the fitted line. The mathematical model for EWR of EDM on molybdenum high-speed steel material and the considered process variables was obtained within 95% confidence interval after reducing the not significant terms as follows:

$$ROC = +0.073 +5.389E\text{-}003*A +4.944E\text{-}003*B \tag{1.19}$$

where: A is peak current IP and B, ON-time.

1.29.2 INTERACTION PLOT FOR ROC OF EDM ON MHSS

Figure 1.33 presents the interaction plot of IP, ON-time, and gap voltage on ROC shows that there is interaction effect of parameters on ROC. An interaction effect of parameters on ROC happened when the effect of one parameter changes depending on the level of another parameter as it can be analyzed that there is an interaction effect of machining parameters on the Ra. This is because the three machining parameters IP, ON-time, and gap voltage determine the size of discharge energy.

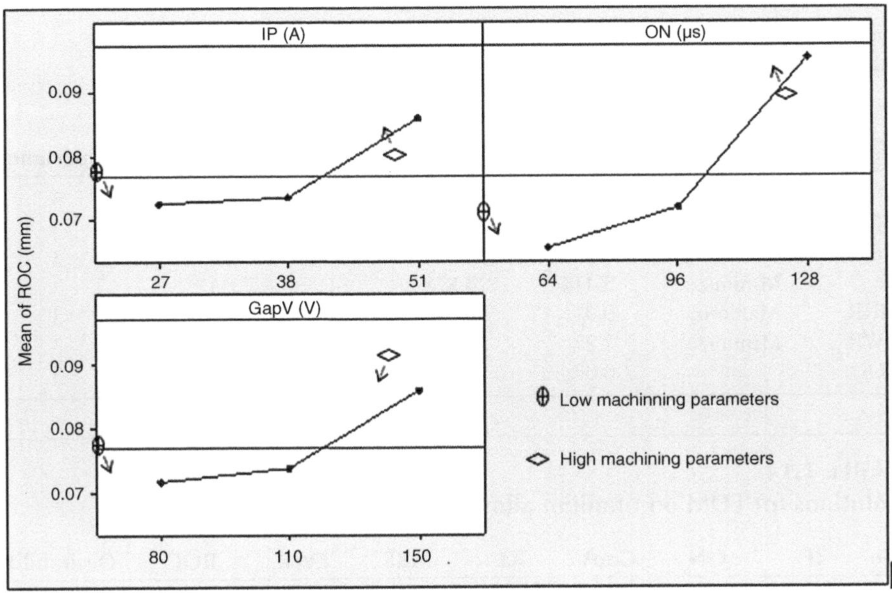

FIGURE 1.32   Effects plot for ROC of EDM on MHSS.

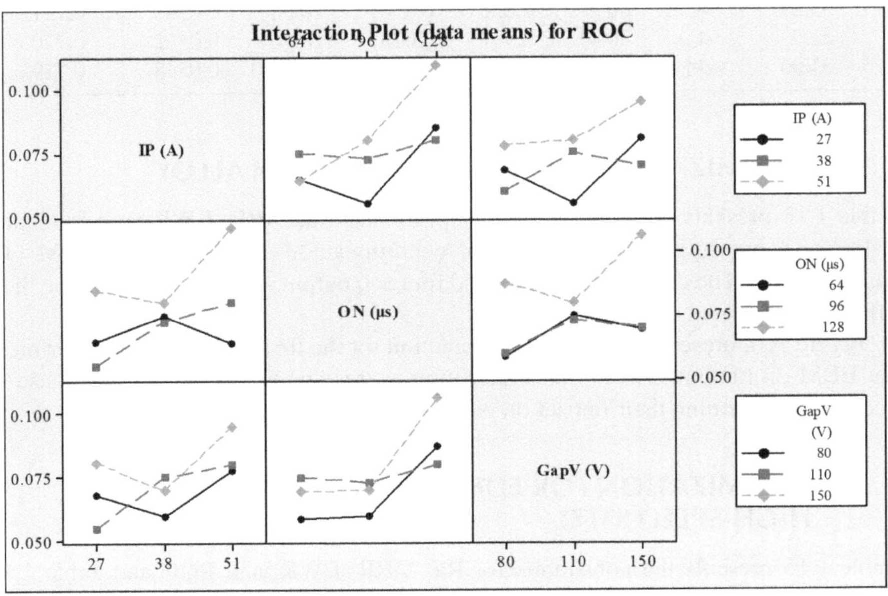

FIGURE 1.33   Interaction plot for ROC of EDM on MHSS.

TABLE 1.13
Parameter constraints for EDM on titanium alloy

Name	Goal	Low	High	Lower weight	Upper weight	Importance
IP	In range	27	51	1	1	3
ON		64	128	1	1	3
GapV		80	150	1	1	3
Ra	Minimize	5.414	14.828	1	1	3
MRR	Maximize	0.01	0.042	1	1	3
EWR	Minimize	7.27	55.556	1	1	3
ROC		0.03	0.112	1	1	3

TABLE 1.14
Solutions for EDM on titanium alloy

No	IP	ON	GapV	Ra	MRR	EWR	ROC	Desirability
1	33.37	64	80	7.069	0.0303	18.49	0.0563	0.7223
2	33.5	64	80	7.097	0.0304	18.55	0.0564	0.7222
3	33.18	64	80	7.030	0.0301	18.41	0.0562	0.7222
4	32.9	64	80	6.971	0.0298	18.28	0.0560	0.7221
5	34.13	64	80	7.229	0.0310	18.84	0.0568	0.7218
6	33.21	64.36	80	7.056	0.0301	18.58	0.0560	0.7215
7	32.97	64	80.41	6.999	0.0297	18.36	0.0562	0.7203
8	31.35	64	80	6.648	0.0280	17.59	0.0548	0.7193

1.30   OPTIMIZATION FOR EDM ON TITANIUM ALLOY

Table 1.13 presents the constraints for optimizing Ra, MRR, EWR, and ROC and Table 1.14 presents the optimal set of conditions for experiment OF EDM ON titanium alloy. The criteria were indicated for each output response to determine their effect on individual desirability.

Figure 1.34 presents the desirability function for the first solution in an experiment for EDM on titanium alloy. Goals and limits were established for each response to accurately determine their impact on overall desirability.

1.31   OPTIMIZATION FOR EDM ON MOLYBDENUM HIGH-SPEED STEEL

Table 1.15 presents the constraints for Ra, MRR, EWR, and ROC and Table 1.16 presents the optimal set of conditions with higher desirability function required for obtaining desired response characteristics under specified constraints The criteria were indicated for each output response to determine their effect on individual desirability.

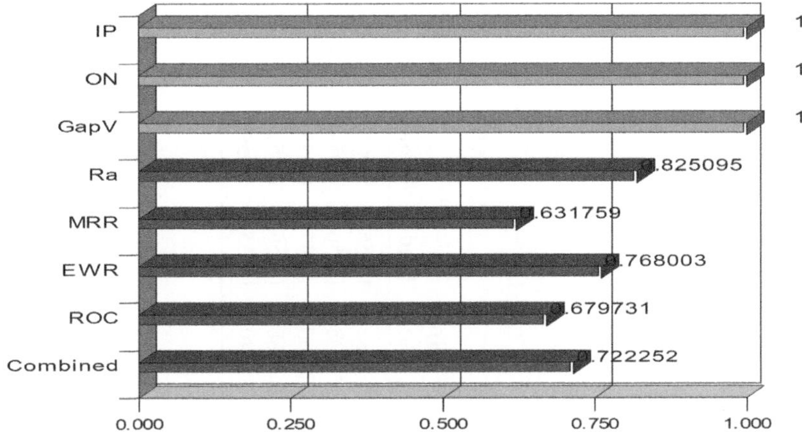

FIGURE 1.34 Desirability for EDM on titanium alloy.

TABLE 1.15
Parameter constraints for EDM on MHSS

Name	Goal	Low	High	Lower weight	Upper weight	Importance
IP	In range	27	51	1	1	3
ON		64	128	1	1	3
GapV		80	150	1	1	3
Ra	Minimize	7.241	17.759	1	1	3
MRR	Maximize	0.057475	0.556164	1	1	3
EWR	Minimize	0.497512	6	1	1	3
ROC		0.045	0.135	1	1	3

TABLE 1.16
Solutions for EDM on MHSS

No	IP	ON	GapV	Ra	MRR	EWR	ROC	Desirability
1	40.76	67.28	80	11.525	0.2744	2.324	0.063	0.6072
2	40.69	67.85	80	11.529	0.2744	2.313	0.064	0.6072
3	40.86	67.55	80	11.553	0.2757	2.322	0.064	0.6072
4	40.79	66.28	80	11.505	0.273	2.343	0.063	0.6072
5	40.44	68.54	80	11.498	0.2726	2.295	0.064	0.6071
6	39.92	72.88	80	11.518	0.2717	2.219	0.065	0.6064
7	41.7	70.93	80	11.813	0.2869	2.300	0.065	0.6062
8	37.84	88.74	80	11.551	0.2668	2.084	0.069	0.5975
9	34.66	111.76	150	12.306	0.3011	2.214	0.082	0.5647
10	34.66	111.42	150	12.295	0.3007	2.224	0.082	0.5647
11	35.06	110.71	150	12.354	0.3039	2.239	0.082	0.5646
12	35.7	104.75	150	12.315	0.3044	2.422	0.080	0.5635

TABLE 1.17
Validation test for EDM on titanium alloy

No	IP	ON	GapV	Ra			MRR			EWR			ROC		
				Pred	Actual	Error (%)	Pred	Actual	Error (%)	Pred	Actual	Error (%)	Pred	Actual	Error (%)
1	33.37	64	80	7.069	7.512	5.89	0.030	0.028	-6.93	18.492	19.235	3.86	0.056	0.061	8.11
4	32.9	64	80	6.971	7.235	3.65	0.030	0.027	-9.12	18.278	18.724	2.38	0.056	0.058	3.23
5	34.13	64	80	7.229	7.462	3.12	0.031	0.034	8.98	18.843	18.365	-2.60	0.057	0.055	-3.89
7	32.97	64	80.41	6.999	6.674	-4.86	0.030	0.028	-7.39	18.360	17.846	-2.88	0.056	0.052	-8.23
8	31.35	64	80	6.648	6.728	1.19	0.028	0.029	4.64	17.591	17.84	1.40	0.055	0.059	7.93

TABLE 1.18
Validation test for EDM on MHSS

No	IP	ON	GapV	Ra			MRR			EWR			ROC		
				Pred	Actual	Error (%)	Pred	Actual	Error (%)	Pred	Actual	Error (%)	Pred	Actual	Error (%)
1	40.76	67.28	80	11.520	10.763	-7.03	0.274	0.302	9.12	2.324	2.512	7.46	0.064	0.071	10.23
2	40.69	67.85	80	11.530	11.021	-4.62	0.274	0.301	8.83	2.313	2.175	-6.35	0.064	0.071	9.18
7	41.7	70.93	80	11.813	12.554	5.90	0.287	0.2662	-7.81	2.300	2.563	10.24	0.066	0.060	-9.36
8	37.84	88.74	80	11.551	12.801	9.76	0.267	0.2972	10.21	2.084	2.282	8.68	0.070	0.071	2.06
9	34.66	111.76	150	12.306	13.237	7.03	0.301	0.2847	-5.78	2.214	2.437	9.14	0.082	0.075	-9.39

1.32 VALIDATION TEST

Validation tests were run with some selected predicted machining parameters setting to test at the optimal factor's levels. Tables 1.17 and 1.18 present the validation test for PM-EDM on titanium alloy and molybdenum high-speed steel and for PM-EDM of molybdenum high-speed steel. Five confirmation experiments have been conducted at the optimum settings of the process parameters. Analyses of the validation experiments show that the actual values of Ra, MRR, TWR, and OC are within 95% of the prediction interval. Due to error percentage which is, in most cases, less than 10%, it can conclude that indicates that the empirical models developed in this work are reasonably reliable for prediction of Ra, MRR, TWR, and OC with a respective acceptable error.

1.33 CONCLUSIONS

In this research, it is established that the use of PM-EDM improves the surface quality on titanium alloy for biomedical and industrial applications. PM-EDM reduces the surface roughness, micro-cracks, craters, and voids on the machined surface. This is attributed due to transfer of alloying elements deposited and uniform distribution of particles from nano aluminum onto the machined surface. The created carbon enriched surface layer also improves osseointegration of the titanium alloy workpiece.

Experiments were run using a designed and fabricated PM-EDM open system.

1. The new PM-EDM open system was successfully designed, fabricated, tested, and analyzed.

    Ra, MRR, EWR, and ROC of nano aluminum PM-EDM on titanium are, respectively, 38.46% reduced, 40% increased, 17.39% reduced, and 16.66% reduced as compared to Ra, MRR, EWR, and ROC of conventional EDM on titanium alloy.

2. Ra, MRR, EWR, and ROC of nano aluminum PM-EDM on molybdenum high-speed steel are, respectively, 16.21% reduced, 17.5% increased, 37.77% reduced, and 16.66% reduced as compared to Ra, MRR, EWR, and ROC of conventional EDM.

3. Nano tungsten PM-EDM on molybdenum high-speed steel is slightly improved with Ra which is about 10.8% reduced; EWR and ROC are reduced about 16.66% and 9.1%, respectively, as compared to conventional EDM on molybdenum high-speed steel.

4. Tungsten PM-EDM with surfactant of molybdenum high-speed steel is not much improved as compared to EDM and PM-EDM of molybdenum high-speed steel.

5. The use of nano aluminum in PM-EDM on titanium alloy and molybdenum high-speed steel results in good output results as compared to nano tungsten powder PM-EDM.

6. PM-EDM marginally enhanced corrosion rate on titanium alloy due to the deposited and embedment of nano aluminum on machined surface. Corrosion is 41.97% reduced when using aluminum PM-EDM on titanium alloy as

compared to corrosion of conventional EDM on titanium alloy. PM-EDM is explored to have potential in biomedical and industry applications.

7. Generate the mathematical models and statistical analysis of output responses namely surface roughness, MRR, EWR subjected to EDM input machining parameters.

8. Synthesize the optimal PM-EDM and EDM parameters on titanium alloy and molybdenum high-speed tool steel using nano aluminum and nano tungsten.

REFERENCES

[1] E. C. Jameson, *Electrical discharge machining*. Society of Manufacturing Engineers, Dearbern, MI, 2001.

[2] H. El-Hofy, *Advanced machining processes: nontraditional and hybrid machining processes*. McGraw Hill Professional, New York, 2005.

[3] M. Gostimirovic, P. Kovac, M. Sekulic, and B. Skoric, "Influence of discharge energy on machining characteristics in EDM," *J. Mech. Sci. Technol.*, vol. 26, no. 1, pp. 173–179, 2012.

[4] E. B. Guitrau, *"The electrical discharge machining handbook,"* ed: Hanser Gardner Publications, Cincinnati, 1997.

[5] H. A. Youssef and H. El-Hofy, *Machining technology: machine tools and operations*. CRC Press, Boca Raton, FL, 2008.

[6] S. F. Miller, C.-C. Kao, A. J. Shih, and J. Qu, "Investigation of wire electrical discharge machining of thin cross-sections and compliant mechanisms," *Int. J. Machine Tools Manufact.*, vol. 45, no. 15, pp. 1717–1725, 2005.

[7] A. Khanra, L. Pathak, and M. Godkhindi, "Application of new tool material for electrical discharge machining (EDM)," *Bull. Mater. Sci.*, vol. 32, no. 4, pp. 401–405, 2009.

[8] S. Daneshmand, E. F. Kahrizi, A. A. L. Neyestanak, and M. M. Ghahi, "Experimental investigations into electro discharge machining of NiTi shape memory alloys using rotational tool," *Int. J. Electrochem. Sci.*, vol. 8, pp. 7484–7497, 2013.

[9] J. Stráský, M. Janeček, P. Harcuba, M. Bukovina, and L. Wagner, "The effect of microstructure on fatigue performance of Ti–6Al–4V alloy after EDM surface treatment for application in orthopaedics," *J. Mech. Behav. Biomed. Mater.*, vol. 4, no. 8, pp. 1955–1962, 2011.

[10] J. Stráský, J. Havlíková, L. Bačáková, P. Harcuba, M. Mhaede, and M. Janeček, "Characterization of electric discharge machining, subsequent etching and shot-peening as a surface treatment for orthopedic implants," *Appl. Surf. Sci.*, vol. 281, pp. 73–78, 2013.

[11] G. Manivasagam, D. Dhinasekaran, and A. Rajamanickam, "Biomedical implants: corrosion and its prevention-a review," *Recent Patents Corros. Sci.*, vol. 2, no. 1, pp. 40–54, 2010.

[12] S.-L. Chen, M.-H. Lin, C.-C. Chen, and K.-L. Ou, "Effect of electro-discharging on formation of biocompatible layer on implant surface," *J. Alloys Cpds.*, vol. 456, no. 1, pp. 413–418, 2008.

[13] A. Hasçalık and U. Çaydaş, "Electrical discharge machining of titanium alloy (Ti–6Al–4V)," *Appl. Surf. Sci.*, vol. 253, no. 22, pp. 9007–9016, 2007.

[14] M. Kiyak and O. Cakır, "Examination of machining parameters on surface roughness in EDM of tool steel," *J. Mater. Process. Technol.*, vol. 191, no. 1, pp. 141–144, 2007.

[15] Y. Guu, H. Hocheng, C. Chou, and C. Deng, "Effect of electrical discharge machining on surface characteristics and machining damage of AISI D2 tool steel," *Mater. Sci. Eng. A,* vol. 358, no. 1, pp. 37–43, 2003.

[16] Y. Guu and M. T.-K. Hou, "Effect of machining parameters on surface textures in EDM of Fe-Mn-Al alloy," *Mater. Sci. Eng. A,* vol. 466, no. 1, pp. 61–67, 2007.

[17] A. Krishna, G. S. B. Uyyala, and Kumar, A, (2014). "Performance analysis of electrical discharge machining parameters on RENE 80 nickel super alloy using statistical tools." *Int. J. Mach. Machinab. Mater.2, 15*(3–4), 212–234..

[18] ASME Standard, "B46. 1-2002," *Surface texture (Surface roughness, waviness, and lay),* The American Society of Mechanical Engineers, An American National Standard, New York, pp. 1–98, 2002.

[19] P. Harcuba, L. Bačáková, J. Stráský, M. Bačáková, K. Novotná, and M. Janeček, "Surface treatment by electric discharge machining of Ti–6Al–4V alloy for potential application in orthopaedics," *J. Mech. Behav. Biomed. Mater.,* vol. 7, pp. 96–105, 2012.

[20] Y.-Y. Tsai and T. Masuzawa, "An index to evaluate the wear resistance of the electrode in micro-EDM," *J. Mater. Process. Technol.,* vol. 149, no. 1, pp. 304–309, 2004.

[21] E. Garba,, A. M. Abdul-Rani, N. A. Yunus, A. A. A. Aliyu, I. A Gul, M. Al-Amin, and R. Aliyu, (2023). A review of electrode manufacturing methods for electrical discharge machining: current status and future perspectives for surface alloying. *Machines, 11*(9), 906.

[22] P. N. Singh, K. Raghukandan, M. Rathinasabapathi, and B. Pai, "Electric discharge machining of Al–10% SiC$_P$ as-cast metal matrix composites," *J. Mater. Process. Technol.,* vol. 155, pp. 1653–1657, 2004.

[23] P. N. Singh, K. Raghukandan, M. Rathinasabapathi, and B. Pai, "Electric discharge machining of Al–10% SiC p as-cast metal matrix composites," *J. Mater. Process. Technol.,* vol. 155, pp. 1653–1657, 2004.

[24] E. Astm, *"384." Standard test method for microhardness of materials,"* American Society for Testing and Materials ASTM, Annual Book of Standards, West Conshohocken, PA, vol. 3, 1999.

[25] L. Tarasov and N. Thibault, "Determination of Knoop hardness numbers independent of load," *Trans. ASM,* vol. 38, pp. 331–353, 1947.

[26] H. Sidhom, F. Ghanem, T. Amadou, G. Gonzalez, and C. Braham, "Effect of electro discharge machining (EDM) on the AISI316L SS white layer microstructure and corrosion resistance," *Int. J. Adv. Manufact. Technol.,* vol. 65, no. 1–4, pp. 141–153, 2013.

[27] A. Casagrande, G. Cammarota, and L. Micele, "Relationship between fatigue limit and Vickers hardness in steels," *Mater. Sci. Eng. A,* vol. 528, no. 9, pp. 3468–3473, 2011.

2 PM-EDM of Titanium and Molybdenum Alloys

Alexis Mouangue Nanimina, Ahmad Majdi Abdul-Rani, Elhuseini Garba, and Saeed Rubaiee

2.1 INTRODUCTION

2.1.1 Hybrid EDM

Hybrid-electrical discharge machining (EDM) processes involve combination of at least two different types of energy to improve the conventional EDM. Employing ultrasonic vibration to the electrode or workpiece, gas–liquid mixture, rotating disc electrode, and powder-mixed dielectric fluid are some of the methods applied to improve the EDM performance on difficult to machine materials.

2.1.2 Dry-EDM

Dry-EDM uses a gas–liquid mixture at high-pressure supplied through a thin-walled pipe. The gas removes the debris from the spark gap and cools down the workpiece and electrode. Helium and argon can be used as a dielectric fluid medium to drill holes using copper electrodes. Kunieda and Yoshida [1] carried out research on EDM in gas using oxygen when machining steel (S45C) with copper–tungsten (Cu–W) electrode. The result shows that the material remove rate (MRR) and electrode wear ratio (EWR) are improved with increased oxygen concentrations. Kunieda et al. [2] did another study on high-speed 3D milling cavities using dry EDM. Mild steel (SS400) was used as workpiece material and copper (Cu) as electrode material. The finding shows that high material removal rate (MRR) can be obtained without losing the advantage of the low tool-electrode wear of dry EDM. Whereas, Sreejit and Ngoi [3] stated that dry EDM must be ecologically desirable for manufacturing. The result stated that dry machining requires suitable measures to compensate for the absence of coolants. Thus, need further improvement of dry EDM techniques for implementation in industries. Some other works were carried out by researchers on dry EDM to investigate the performance of EDM [4–8]. From the findings, it can be concluded that dry EDM can improve the MRR and avoid the problem of debris deposition. There is a need for more investigation on other output responses to establish the use of dry EDM.

DOI: 10.1201/9781003456018-2

2.1.3 Ultrasonic Vibration EDM

The use of a vibratory wave of frequency above 16 kilocycles per second (Hz) is another technique. Abrasive slurry is replaced by a suitable dielectric fluid (kerosene, distilled water). In the ultrasonic process, vibration of the tool or workpiece in combination with EDM removes material effectively. Ultrasonic vibrations can provide larger particles, many particles with spherical geometry and more uniformity of spherical and non-spherical particles, uniform mixing of materials and more collision between debris particles. Zhang et al. studied the effect of ultrasonic vibration EDM in gas (UVEDM) [9–11]. They found that UEDM in gas is an effective machining method. The MRR of UVEDM in gas is much higher compared to that of EDM in gas and EDM. Abdullah and Shabgard [12] investigated the effect of ultrasonic vibration combined with EDM on cemented tungsten carbide (WC–Co) using copper electrode vibration. They found that more material was removed at a low peak current and ON-time. Other investigations of ultrasonic vibration-assisted EDM were conducted by some researchers for improvement of EDM [13–15]. Using this technique, the stability of EDM is improved but needs more investigation to establish the implementation.

2.1.4 Rotating Disc Electrode

The rotating disk electrode technique is used to improve the debris removal. The motion and direction of the electrode is generally normal to the work surface. The electrode can be cylindrical (Figure 2.5a) or disk-shaped (Figure 2.5b). The effect of the tool rotation results in fine debris particles and improved process stability. Singh and Pandey [16] reported on EDM of imonic75 superalloy using a rotary copper disk electrode. The results show that the aspect ratio and peak current affect the machining performance the most. Rotating disk electrode easily flushes away the debris causing better machining process.

Chow et al. [17, 18] investigated the use of SiC powder in water as the medium during the micro-slit EDM process. They found that the added SiC powder improved electrical conductivity of the medium and enlarged the gap distance, thus improving the MRR. On the other hand, Chattopadhyay et al. [19] developed a model for rotary EDM when machining copper–steel workpiece materials. Results show that peak current and ON-time are the parameters affecting the MRR and EWR the most.

2.1.5 Magnetic Forced-Assisted EDM

A study on the effects of magnetic force-assisted EDM was carried out by Lin et al. [20] using Taguchi orthogonal array as a fractional factorial design. Peak current and ON-time are the main selected machining parameters on the MRR, EWR, and Ra. Results show a lot of improvement in terms of the MRR, EWR, and Ra.

2.2 POWDER MIXED EDM

For powder-mixed electrical discharge machining (PM-EDM), a metallic powder is mixed with dielectric fluid in a tank. For the circulation of the dielectric fluid, the experimental setup is equipped with a stirring system. PM-EDM circulation system can be employed to enable the reuse of metallic powder. The effects of metallic powder depend mainly on its physical properties, particle size, and powder concentration. The metallic powders used in this research are nano aluminum and nano tungsten and the main characteristics to consider when selecting metallic powders are as follows:

Electrical conductivity: metallic powder with high or good conductivity will easily promote more electrons to ionize or breakdown the dielectric fluid for quicker creation of electrical discharge which flows widely in EDM area.

Thermal conductivity: high thermal conductivity of metallic powder will easily dissipate heat from machining area to the dielectric fluid.

Density: low density of metallic powder will contribute to the suspension of powder in dielectric.

Melting: low melting point will contribute to the melting of metallic powder to be deposited and bounded with machined surface for improving its characteristics.

Powder size: fine metallic powder improves machining rates, gives lowest wear ratio and surface roughness. Metallic powder grain size can be classified as very coarse (>1000 µm); coarse (355–1000 µm); moderately fine (180–355 µm), fine (125–180 µm), and very fine (90–125 µm) and the particle shapes can be acicular, angular, granular, and spherical [21].

Powder concentration: the amount of metallic powder in the dielectric fluid will promote more electrons to be energized, contributing to the fast breakdown of dielectric fluid and evenly distribution of electrical discharge. Many researchers analyzed that optimal metallic powder concentration improves EDM machining performance.

2.2.1 PRINCIPLE OF PM-EDM

The operating principle of PM-EDM involves the steps described as follows:

Metallic powder is added to dielectric fluid, and it fills up the gap between the electrode and workpiece. When potential difference is applied between the electrode and workpiece, an electric field between 105 and 107 V/m will be generated. Metallic powder particles under the machining zone get energized and form a bridge between the electrode and workpiece The energy of the conductive particle promotes the breakdown of dielectric fluid and increases the gap between the electrode and workpiece. Hence, early discharges start under the electrode area and create fast sparks which erode the workpiece. The presence of metallic powder ensures uniform distribution of spark, and the electrical density of the spark decreases which reduces craters, cracks, and voids on machined surface. Some researchers found that accumulation of sparks between two consecutive metallic powder particles in machining area results in series of discharges [22–26]. This increases the sparking intensity within discharges leading to faster erosion from the workpiece, and therefore increases MRR.

2.2.2 RECENT DEVELOPMENT IN **PM-EDM**

The PM-EDM process involves the use of different types of conductive or semi-conductive powders mixed with dielectric fluid in attempt to improve the EDM performance [27, 28]. Table 2.1 presents some research in PM-EDM. Metallic powder suspended in EDM dielectric fluid is another means of improving the machined surface properties. PM-EDM facilitates EDM ignition phases creating higher discharge leading to low dielectric fluid breakdown strength [35, 36–38]. Some other works were performed by some researchers in PM-EDM seeking for establishment of these techniques [39–41].

TABLE 2.1
Research on PM-EDM

Authors/ Reference	Work material	Powder/size	Output measures	Remarks
Uno et al. (2001)[29]	Alloy tool steel SKD61	Carbon, nickel/ 5 μm	Coated composition, Ra, hardness, wear resistance	Ra in nickel PM-EDM is smaller than that in conventional EDM. The deposit of nickel on EDM machined surface becomes larger with an increase of nickel concentration. EDM machined surface with nickel PM-EDM becomes harder than that in conventional EDM due to TiC embedded on the machined surface.
Chow et al. (2000)[30]	Ti-6Al-4V/ Copper	SiC, aluminum/ 1 μm	Gap distance, MRR, Ra	SiC removes more material than Al in PMDM. SiC induces a lot of hardness. SiC reacts with carbon particles embedded on the machined surface and on the area of the electrode. It has been found that Al powder is the best among the selected powders due to its optimal conductivity and light weight.

TABLE 2.1 (Continued)
Research on PM-EDM

Authors/ Reference	Work material	Powder/size	Output measures	Remarks
Pecas et al. (2008)[31]	AISI H13/ Cu, 1, 9, 16, 32, and 64 cm²	Si/10μm	Surface topography, Ra, white-layer	PM-EDM reduces the Ra, crater, and white-layer size. Electrode areas influence the quality of the machined surface causing degradation of the electrode and workpiece surfaces.
Soumyakant et al (2012)[32]	EN 31 steel/Cu, 25 mm	Silicon/ 20–30 μm	MRR, Ra	Use of PM-EDM promotes reduction of the Ra and improves the MRR. Mathematical models for prediction of the MRR and SR through four process parameters.
Kumar and Batra (2012) [33]	OHNS O2 die steel, HC-HCr D2 die steel, H13 die steel/ Copper	Tungsten/30–40 μm	Surface analysis, optimum machining parameters	A certain amount of material was transferred from the powder to the machined surface. The presence of tungsten carbide was found. The embedded tungsten carbide improves the micro-hardness of the machined surface.
Kansal et al. (2005)[34]	EN-31 tool steel/Cu, Ø25m	/Si, 20–30 μm	MRR, Ra	Silicon PMDM affects both the MRR and SR. The MRR is increased when the concentration of silicon is increased. The result shows improvement in the Ra with an additive of silicon powder.

2.2.3 PM-EDM Operating System

During the PM-EDM process, the use of powder-mixed with a dielectric fluid can be performed directly in the original tank of the EDM or in a separate tank. The use of the original tank requires more than 80 l of dielectric fluid. The concern with the use of original tank of EDM is that a large amount of metallic powder is needed to be added to the dielectric fluid, and the mixed powder dielectric fluid circulates through the original EDM circulation and filtering systems. This might easily damage the filtering system and it wastes the dielectric fluid and economically, it is not profitable [35, 42].

From the literature review, most of the researchers have employed metallic powder in a separate tank placed in the original tank of EDM and there is no connection between the operating tank and original EDM tank [35, 43]. The separated tank is mainly called an operating tank or machining tank where machining is performed. The machine setup is made of a small tank and equipped with or without a stirrer. Use of a stirrer is to ensure the uniform distribution of the metallic powder. The operating tank so far described in literature can be totally isolated from or connected to a supply reservoir. This section aims to categorize the two main operating tanks.

2.2.4 First Category of Operating System

The first category of the operating tank is the one isolated completely from the existing EDM tank and any other EDM dielectric fluid supply system in this category of tank, powder-mixed with dielectric fluid is contained in the operating tank only. There is no renewal of the dielectric fluid or powder-mixed dielectric fluid. A stirrer can be placed in the operating tank for the uniform mixing of metallic powder. In some cases, a circulating pump is placed to circulate the powder-mixed dielectric fluid inside the operating tank only. This category of tank can be proposed in this research work to be called a "closed PM-EDM system" because there is no contact with the external reservoir for the renewal of the dielectric fluid or the powder-mixed dielectric fluid. Even though a circulating pump is placed in the operating tank, the circulation is in the operating tank only, not in a renewal system. A couple of research have been performed using the close PM-EDM system as presented in Table 2.2.

2.2.5 Second Category of Operating System

The second category of the operating tank is the one connected to any external source or reservoir for renewal of the powder-mixed with the dielectric fluid in this second category of tank, a dielectric fluid circulation and filtering system can be designed for the renewal of the dielectric fluid and reuse of the metallic powder. Therefore, powder-mixed with dielectric fluid can be constantly renewed and the metallic powder can be reused. Stirrers can be placed in the operating tank and the external reservoir for the uniform mixing of the metallic powder. This category of tank can be proposed in this research work to be called an "open PM-EDM system." In this system, with the circulation of the powder-mixed dielectric fluid, there is an advantage, not only to renew the dielectric fluid with the metallic powder but also to filter and separate the metallic powder from the debris and other elements from the machining that can disturb the performance of EDM.

Some research works have been carried out using an open PM-EDM system. Tzeng et al. [47, 48] studied the effects of PM-EDM using an "open operating tank" and explored optimization of PM-EDM. They found that particle size, concentration, and density on the electrical and thermal conductivity are the most important parameters. Since no stirrer was provided in the operating tank or in the mixing tank, the uniformity of the powder-mixed dielectric fluid might not be achieved. Adding a filter in the circulation system can contribute to retaining the debris but provides a suitable size of filter to allow the metallic powder to pass through.

TABLE 2.2
Research on open PM-EDM system

Authors/ Reference	Work material	Powder/size	Output measures	Remarks
Kansal et al. (2007) [35]	AISI D2/Cu	Silicon	MRR	Peak current, ON-time, OFF-time, powder concentration and gain affect the MRR in PM-EDM a lot.
Singh and Yeh (2012) [44]	Aluminum alloy/Cu	SiC	MRR, TWR, and SR	Results show that Peak current, ON-time, OFF-time, gap voltage, Duty cycle, and powder concentration affect the performance characteristics in terms of MRR, TWR and SR
Batish and Bhattachary (2012) [45]	H11 and H13 die steels/ copper, tungsten–copper, and graphite	Graphite, aluminum, copper, tungsten	Micro-hardness, microstructure	Addition of powders to the dielectric fluid affects the micro-hardness and micro-structure. Transfer and deposition of material on the machined surface was analyzed. Micro-hardness of H11 increased by 37% and that of H13 by 56%.
Hu et al. (2011) [46]	Aluminum matrix Composite/ Cu	Aluminum/ 6 µm	MRR, Ra, micro-topography, hardness	PM-EDM has higher surface hardness and wear-resistance, so improves the machined surface properties.

Wong et al. [49] carried out a study on a PM-EDM opened system using silicon, aluminum, graphite, silicon carbide, crushed glass and, molybdenum sulfide. Aluminum powder has been reported to produce a fine surface quality. The concern is the contamination of the whole dielectric fluid that might affect the results since the powder is directed to the tank and the same tank is supplied by the dielectric fluid from the main feed pump which is not mixed with powder. Cogun and Karacay [50] conducted research on the effect of PM-EDM on machining performance in an open operating tank. Mixing graphite powder with a kerosene dielectric fluid improved the surface quality more. Since no stirrer was placed in the operating tank, the concern may be the metallic powder and debris settlement at the bottom of the operating tank.

2.2.6 PM-EDM OF IMPLANTS

Since the limitation in using EDM for machining implants is the fatigue performance due to surface cracks, brittle oxidized surface recast layer, internal tensile stresses, and notch sensitivity of titanium alloys [51], PM-EDM may have potential surface modification for the improvement of implant surface properties and topography, chemical composition and machining rate. Research studies conducted in PM-EDM of implants are limited and need more investigation.

2.3 METHODOLOGY

2.3.1 DESIGN OF EXPERIMENT

A design of experiment (DOE) was done and response surface methodology (RSM) techniques were selected using central composite design (CCD) which has the advantage that certain level adjustments are acceptable. Figure 2.1 presents the flow of DOE procedures. RSM was selected as design technique for this research since the electrical discharge machining process involves many machining parameters. Some machining parameters have interaction effects on output responses. As stated earlier, RSM could analyze the individual and interaction effects of the machining parameters on the responses, and it can predict the most important parameter according to analysis of variance (ANOVA). Depending on where the star points are placed, there are three types of CCD in RSM has three such as circumscribed CCD (CCC), inscribed CCD (CCI), and face-centered CCD (CCF). In CCC, the star points are at some distance alpha (α) from the center based on the properties desired for the design and the number of factors in the design. The star points establish new extremes for the low- and high settings for all factors. Whereas in CCI, the design uses the factor settings as the star points and creates a factorial or fractional factorial design within those limits (in other words, a CCI design is a scaled down CCC design with each factor level of the CCC design divided by α to generate the CCI design). This design also requires five levels of each factor. For CCF design, the star points are at the center of each face of the factorial space, so $\alpha = \pm 1$. This variety requires three levels of each factor [52].

2.3.2 PARAMETERS

Titanium alloy Ti-6Al-4V grade 5, according to ASTM designation B.265-79 and molybdenum high-speed steel specifically SKH51 according to JIS designation, were selected as the workpiece materials. For the specimen preparation, CNC EDM Wire-cut machine FA10 brand was used to cut the raw material into block shape required for clamping on EDM. Titanium alloys and molybdenum high-speed steel

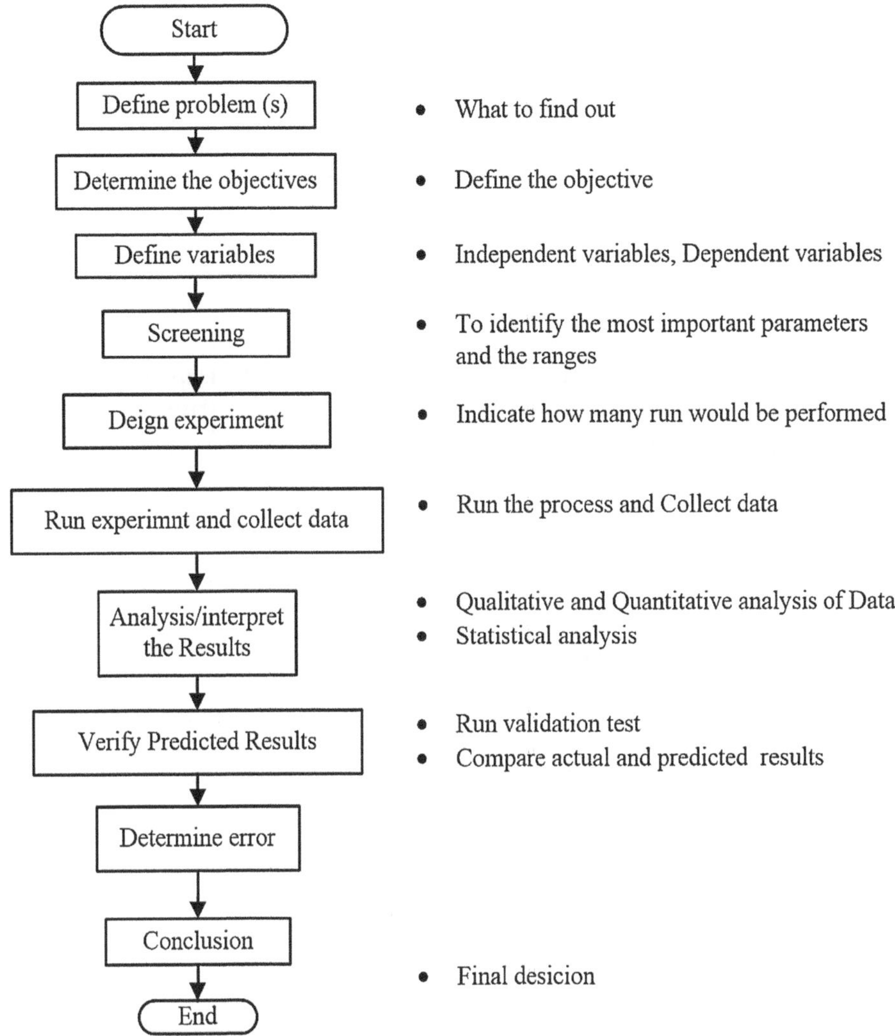

FIGURE 2.1 Flow of experiment procedure.

TABLE 2.3
Composition of molybdenum high-speed steel

Elements	C	Si	Cr	V	W	Mo	Co	Fe
Weight (%)	0.83	0.35	3.75	1.18	1.75	8.70	-	Balance

specimens were prepared to the size of 9 mm × 11 mm × 5 mm for ease of mounting on analysis device requirement. Tables 2.3 and 2.4 present, respectively, the chemical compositions of titanium alloy and molybdenum high-speed steel materials. The properties of the workpiece materials are presented in Table 2.5.

TABLE 2.4
Composition of titanium alloy

Elements	Al	V	Fe	O	C	N	H	Ti
Weight (%)	5.5–6.75	3.5–4.5	≤0.40	≤0.20	≤0.080	≤0.050	≤0.015	87.6–91

TABLE 2.5
Properties of workpiece materials

Materials	Melting Point (°C)	Density (g/cm³)	Young modulus (GPa)	Thermal conductivity (W/m.K)	Hardness (HB)	Electrical resistivity ($\times 10^{-7}$ Ωm)
Molybdenum high-speed steel	1082.0	7.72-8	190-210	19.0	111.0	0.6
Titanium alloy	1660	4.43	120	7.3	334	7.36

TABLE 2.6
Copper–tungsten (W70Cu30) properties

Material	Melting point (°C)	Density (g/cm³)	Young modulus (N/mm²)	Hardness (HV)	Thermal conductivity (W/mK)	Electrical resistivity ($\times 10^{-7}$ Ωcm)
W70Cu30	3410	14.3	225 x 10³	175	154	7.27

2.3.3 ELECTRODE MATERIAL

Cu–W (W70Cu30) was used as electrode material with cross-section of 9 mm × 9 mm. The selection of Cu–W is due to good conductivity of copper and good melting point of tungsten. High electrical conductivity of electrode promotes more electrons from electrode since electric current is the "cutting tool" and high melting point of electrode contributes low wear ratio since EDM is a thermal process. The combination of Cu–W gives optimal electrical and thermal conductivities to the electrode. Table 2.6 presents copper and Cu–W properties.

A square section 9 mm × 9 mm of electrodes was to machine a U-shape workpiece as shown in Figure 2.2.

2.4 PM-EDM METALLIC POWDER

Nano aluminum and nano tungsten powders were selected, and each is mixed separately with dielectric fluid during PM-EDM. The selection of metallic powder was done by considering the expected contribution of metallic powder to the PM-EDM

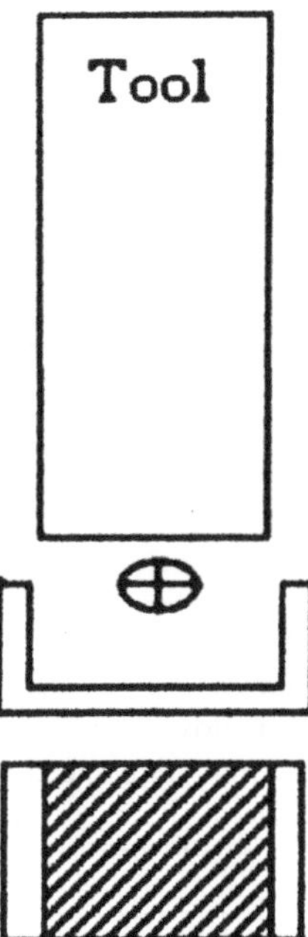

FIGURE 2.2   Cross-section of electrode position and workpiece U shape.

TABLE 2.7
Properties of selected powders

Powder	Melting point (°C)	Density (kg/m^3)	Thermal conductivity (W m^{-1} K^{-1})	Electrical resistivity (10.E6 Siemens/m)	Powder grain size
Aluminum	660	2700	238	36.9	40nm
Tungsten	19000	4500	174	8.9	

process in terms of electrical conductivity, thermal conductivity, density, and melting point properties. From review and compilation of metallic powders, a list of top 10 was made according to each of the properties mentioned above. Thus, nano aluminum and nano tungsten powders were selected. The properties of nano aluminum and nano tungsten powders are presented in Table 2.7.

2.5   PM-EDM PROCESS PARAMETERS

The PM-EDM process parameters such as gap voltage, peak current, ON-time, OFF-time, nano aluminum and nano tungsten concentration, and their ranges are selected based on extensive literature review, pilot study, and the setup range available on

TABLE 2.8
PMEDEM process parameters

Identified variable machining parameters	Symbol	Identified units	Identified range
Gap voltage	GapV	V	80–150
Peak current	IP	A	27–55
ON-time	ON	µs	16–128
OFF-time	OFF	µs	128
Powder types	Nano aluminum		
	Nano tungsten		
Powder grain size	40 nm		
Powder concentration	Pcon	g/l	1–3
Surfactant type	Tween80		
Surfactant concentration	Surfactant	g/l	3
Workpiece types	Titanium alloy		
	Molybdenum high-speed steel		
Depth of cut	DOC	mm	3

TABLE 2.9
Different categories of experiments

No	Experiments	Category
1	**Experiment 1**	Development, testing, and analysis of new PM-EDM system
2	**Experiment 2**	Nano aluminum PM-EDM on Ti-4Al-6V grade 5 titanium alloy
3	**Experiment 3**	Nano aluminum PM-EDM of molybdenum high-speed steel SKH51
4	**Experiment 4**	Nano tungsten PM-EDM of molybdenum high-speed steel SKH51
5	**Experiment 5**	Surfactant and nano tungsten PM-EDM on molybdenum high-speed steel SKH51 on surface roughness (Ra) and material removal rate (MRR)

the EDM machine. These machining parameters are the most general and frequently chosen by researchers [40]. The identified and analyzed most significant process parameters are presented in Table 2.8.

2.6 EXPERIMENTS

The summary of the different categories of experiments is presented in Table 2.10.

- ***Experiment 1:*** experiment consists of development of new PM-EDM circulation system.
- ***Experiment 2***: for Experiment 1, nano aluminum was mixed with EDM dielectric in the PM-EDM system machining Ti-4Al-6V grade 5 titanium alloy workpiece. A total of 30 runs were done according to the DOE template.

TABLE 2.10
Hank´s solution chemical composition: simulated body fluid

Component	NaCl	KCl	$CaCl_2$
	Sodium chloride	Potassium chloride	Calcium chloride
(g/L)	8.00	0.40	0.14
Component	$NaHCO_3$	$MgCl_2.6H_2O$	$MgSO_4.7H2O$
	Sodium bicarbonate	Magnesium chloride hexahydrate	Magnesium sulfate heptahydrate
(g/L)	0.35	0.60	0.06
Component	Na_2HPO_4	KH_2PO_4	Glucose.2H2O
	Sodium phosphate dibasic	Potassium phosphate monobasic	
(g/L)	0.06	0.60	1.0
Component	pH		
(g/L)	6.8		

- ***Experiment 3:*** experiment 4 consisted of mixing nano aluminum dielectric fluid in PM-EDM on molybdenum high-speed steel SKH51.
- ***Experiment 4*** For experiment 5, nano tungsten was mixed with dielectric fluid PM-EDM of molybdenum high-speed steel.
- ***Experiment 5:*** experiment 7 consisted of surfactant and nano tungsten mixed with dielectric fluid in PM-EDM of industrial grade molybdenum high-speed steel in terms of surface roughness and MRR.

2.7 OUTPUT RESPONSES

The output responses investigated in this research such as surface roughness, surface morphology, phase analysis, micro-hardness, fatigue performance, MRR, EWR, and radial overcut (ROC) are presented and described as follows.

2.8 RESULTS

2.8.1 SURFACE ROUGHNESS MEASUREMENT

Surface roughness average (Ra), defined in ASME B46.1-2002 [53], was selected. Measurements were performed on all samples using surface roughness tester Ra is an important parameter used in manufacturing to measure the texture of machined surface which characterizes the quality of the machined surface of a product. Part that has good Ra improves the fatigue performance and corrosion resistance [54]. However, roughness of biomedical implants can contribute to adhesion between the implant and a living bone [55], with rougher surface providing better adhesion but can be detrimental towards resistance to corrosion and fatigue. Craters, voids, and micro-cracks on implant surface reduce their fatigue and corrosion resistance [40]. The measurements were done according to standard ISO 3274:1996 for the nominal characteristics of contact (Stylus) instruments. Three different measurement lines were taken, and an average calculated. The stylus traverses the surface peaks and valleys, and the vertical motion of the stylus is converted by the transducer into an electrical signal which will be analyzed by digital or analog technique. The result in digital profile is stored in a computer and can be analyzed. Sample length was 6 mm, and the cut-off length was 2.5 mm.

2.8.2   MATERIAL REMOVAL RATE

MRR is an important parameter selected to estimate the volume of material removed during a specific time of EDM machining process. MRR is a parameter that describes the least machining cycle time to increase productivity. MRR in grams per minute is the difference of the mass in grams of the workpiece before and after machining to the machining time in minutes. Equation (2.1) was used to determine MRR.

$$MRR = \frac{Mass\,loss\,of\,workpiece}{machining\ time} \tag{2.1}$$

The mass loss is measured by weighing the workpiece before and after machining using the electronic balance machine presented. The electronic balance machine is from branch Mettler Toledo ME3002. The maximum weight that can be measured is 500 g with the resolution of 0.01 g.

2.8.3   SURFACE MORPHOLOGY OF MACHINED SURFACE

EDM is an electro-thermal process which can result in rougher or smooth surface machined surface according to machining parameters setting. Surface roughness measurement using profile-meter is limited to quantify the surface in term of deviation from its original form. It is important to study the surface morphology of machined surface to confirm the result from profile-meter in term of image. From the surface morphology image, defects on machined surface can be characterized in terms of cracks, voids, craters, and phase modification which may either be acceptable or rejected depending on application. Specimens were machined using EDM process at various machining parameter settings. Examination of surface morphology of machined surfaces was done on specimens machined at low- and high-machining parameters for each category of experiments. FESEM Zeiss SUPRA 55VP was used to examine and analyze the machined surfaces. FESEM is a microscope that uses electrons to scan in detail the machined surface as compared to optical microscopy which uses light.

During EDM or PM-EDM process, materials can be transferred from electrode to workpiece and vice versa. The transfer material can be deposited and bound on machined surface improving its hardness and roughness. Therefore, it is important to analyze the materials transferred from electrode or nano aluminum and nano tungsten as evidence of the presence of the transfer elements that contribute to the machined surface enhancement. Analysis of material transfer was done using energy dispersive spectroscopy (EDS) attached to FESEM. EDS analysis involves the generation of an X-ray spectrum from the entire scan area of the SEM.

2.8.4 MICRO-HARDNESS

Hardness testing determines the mechanical property of machined components. Hardness is used to estimate the ductility and resistance to wear, fatigue, and tensile strength properties. Hardness may also be shown to correlate to tensile strength and fatigue in many metals. Measurement of micro-hardness was done using micro-hardness tester. ASTM E 384 standard defines and specifies the micro-indentation hardness test method and parameters of materials [56]. Hardness test uses forces in the 1–1000 gf. With the Vickers hardness test, a diamond with top angle of 136° is used. The Vickers hardness parameter is presented in this research project. Tarasov et al. [57] presented in their work, the details of hardness test procedure.

2.8.5 FATIGUE PERFORMANCE

Fatigue is the progressive and localized structural damage that occurs when a material is subjected to cyclic loading. During EDM or PM-EDM, the repeated electric sparks cause fatigue damage [58]. Fatigue damage includes three stages such as crack initiation, crack propagation, and final fracture. Fatigue of material can also be represented by hardness and some authors have established empirical correlation between hardness and fatigue and ultimate strength in steel as shown in Equations (2.2) and 2.3 [59].

$$\sigma_w = 1.6HV \pm 0.1HV \tag{2.2}$$

where: σ_w is fatigue limit in MPa and HV is the Vickers hardness in kgf/mm^2 and

$$\sigma_w = 0.5\sigma_u \tag{2.3}$$

where: σ_u is the ultimate tensile strength of material.
In this study, Equation (2.2) was used to determine the fatigue of the specimen due to specimen shape and steel base material. The shape specimen limits the use of other fatigue testing standards like standard ASTM E606/E606M using rotating cantilever bending fatigue test machine, constant deflection amplitude cantilever bending test machine.

2.8.6 CORROSION TEST

Corrosion analysis is an important parameter indicator for industry and biomedical engineering because corrosion can affect the mechanical properties and biocompatibility of materials. Corrosion analysis was conducted using linear polarization resistance (LPR) test with three electrodes, according to ASTM G3–89, ASTM G59, and ASTM G31. The use of a three-electrode potentiostat with a separate reference and counter electrode allows the potential and the current at the working electrode (WE) to be measured with little or no "interference" or "contribution" from the other electrodes. Potentiate polarization measurements were used to study the effect of corrosion on Ti-6Al-4V. A design with three electrode cell corrosion was used in this study for corrosion testing. The three electrodes are immersed in a simulated body fluid, Hank's solution as presented in Table 3.9 as the electrolyte [60, 61]. The linear LPR method uses a small voltage of about ±20 mV between the electrodes and the current is measured. The LPR was done in 3 h setting time with six reading points. Ecor (mV) was ranging from -10 to 10 mV with scan rate of 10 mV/s and sample area of 0.33 cm².

In LPR method, a small current is applied (few µA) therefore, there will be change in electrode potential and current. The potentiostat will measure the potential current changes, plot the overvoltage versus current, and calculate the slope. The measured resistance is inversely related to the corrosion rate.

2.8.7 SURFACE MORPHOLOGY OF NANO ALUMINUM PM-EDM ON TITANIUM ALLOY

Figure 2.3 shows the morphology of the machined surface PM-EDM at low (Figure 2.20a) and high (Figure 2.20b) parameter conditions as mentioned above. It indicates that the machined surface is smoother after adding nano aluminum as less crack, crater, and void as compared to the surface morphology of conventional EDM on titanium alloy. This is due to the transfer of alloying elements which melted, deposited,

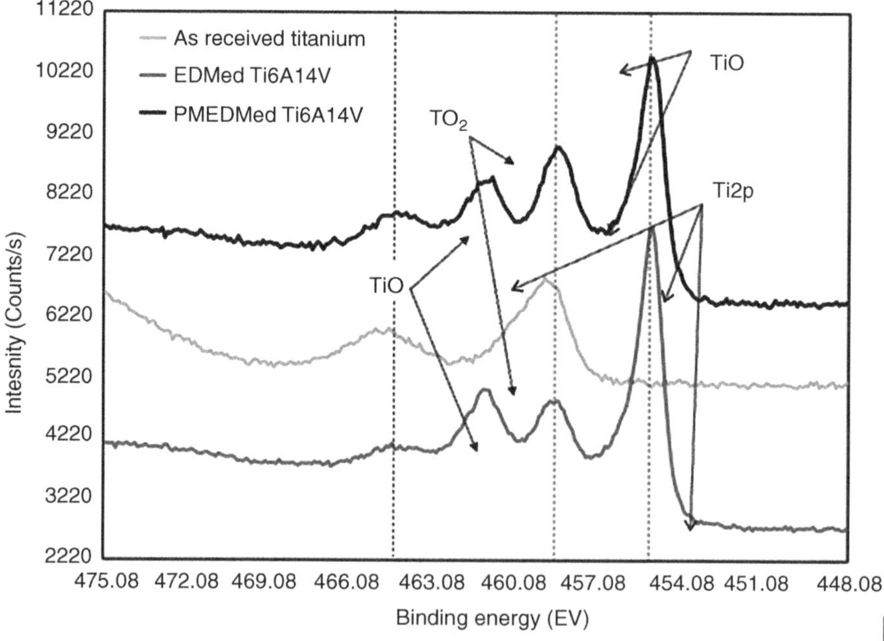

FIGURE 2.3 Morphology of nano aluminum PM-EDM on titanium alloy.

and embedded onto the workpiece machined surface during PM-EDM. The use of nano aluminum mixed with dielectric fluid decreases the presence of micro-cracks on the machined surface as compared to conventional EDM machined surface. The added nano aluminum particles contribute to uniform distribution of discharge energy resulting in small craters, cracks, voids, and globules on the machining surfaces.

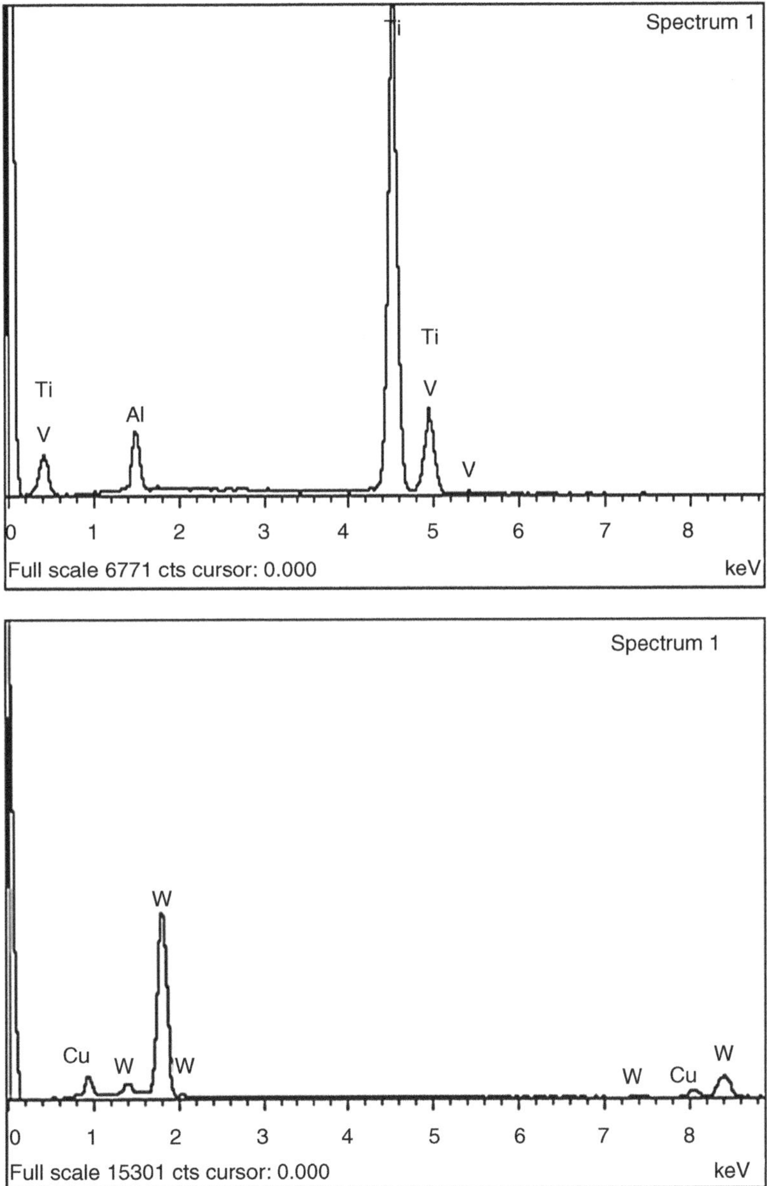

FIGURE 2.4 (a) EDS spectrum of as received titanium alloy workpiece. (b) EDS spectrum of as received copper–tungsten electrode.

EDS spectrum chemical characterization for as received titanium alloy and Cu-W are presented in figure, Figure 2.4a and b, respectively. EDS analysis on EDM machined surfaces both at low machining parameters now clearly indicate the recently embedded carbon, oxygen, copper, and tungsten element previously were not present on the as received titanium alloy workpiece as shown. After nano aluminum PM-EDM on titanium alloy, aluminum, copper, and tungsten elements amounts are increased about 16.33%, 11.24% and 9.10%, respectively, as compared to EDM on titanium alloy.

2.8.8 CORROSION RATE ON TITANIUM ALLOY

The titanium alloy specimens as received and machined using EDM and nano aluminum PM-EDM processes were immersed in Hank´s solution, the body fluid. The results of 3-h LPR with six reading points are presented in Figure 2.5. Ecor (mV)

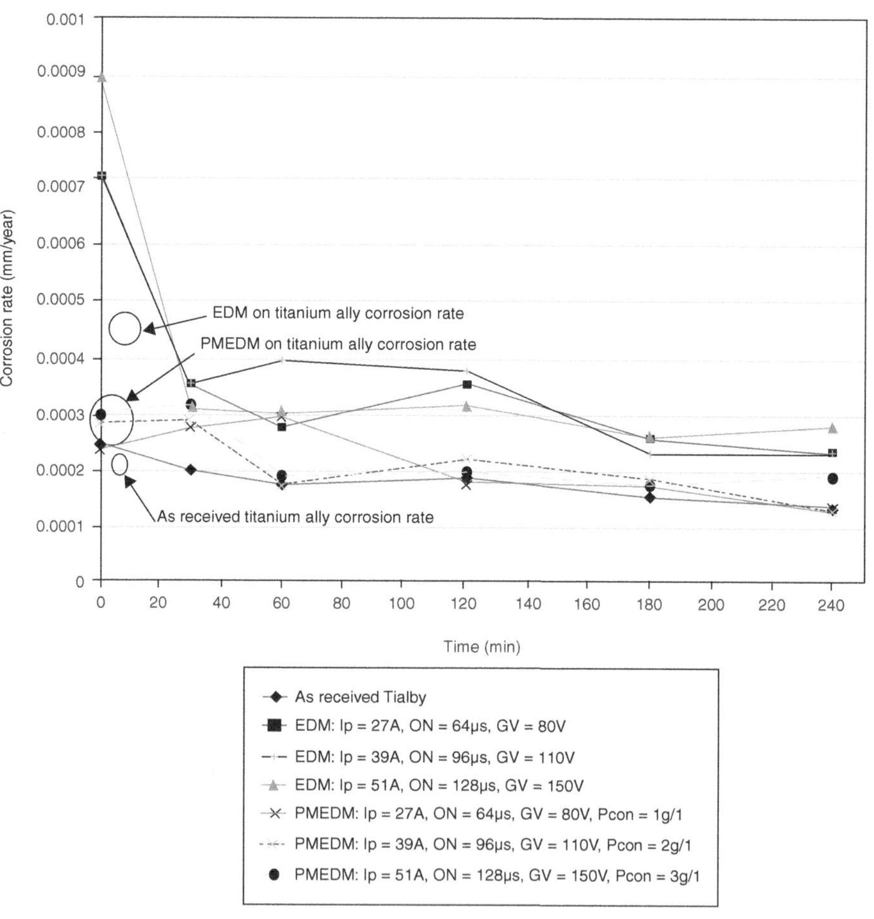

FIGURE 2.5 LPR corrosion rate of EDM and PM-EDM on titanium alloy.

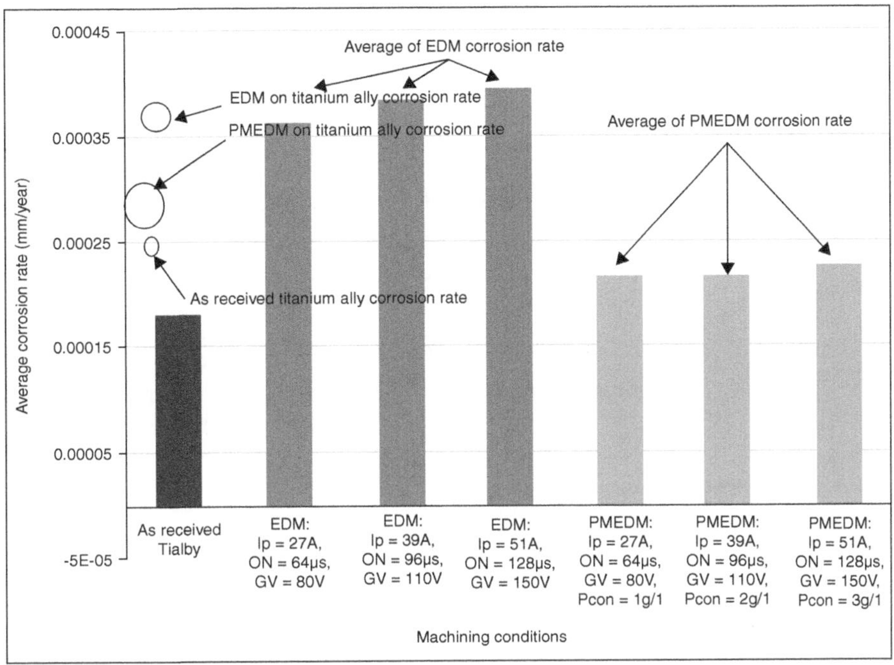

FIGURE 2.6 Average corrosion of as received, EDM and PM-EDM on Ti-6Al-4V.

ranges from -10 to 10 mV with scan rate of 10 mV/s and sample area of 0.33 cm^2. The improvement of the PM-EDM corrosion rate is due to improvement of machined surface irregularities and microstructure by powder-mixed dielectric fluid. Figure 2.6 presents the average corrosion rate of as received, EDM and PM-EDM on titanium alloy. The maximum corrosion rate is found for the conventional EDM on Ti-6Al-4V alloy compared to PM-EDM. The electrochemical corrosion results show that corrosion resistance of the specimens which are machined by EDM is about two times more than the specimens which are machined using PM-EDM. Corrosion is induced during the EDM on titanium alloy, but corrosion rate is reduced with PM-EDM and slightly closer to as received titanium alloy. The average corrosion rate of PM-EDM of 2.28266 × 10^{-4} mm/year on titanium alloy is closed to the accepted corrosion rate for implants which is about 2.5 × 10^{-4} mm/year [62] compared to the average corrosion rate of EDM of 3.98554 × 10^{-4} mm/year. With added nano aluminum, the corrosion of nano aluminum PM-EDM on titanium alloy is reduced to about 41.97%, as compared to the corrosion of conventional EDM on titanium alloy as shown below.

2.8.9 Phase Analysis of Nano Aluminum PM-EDM on Titanium Alloy

XRD was used to examine changes on the nano aluminum PM-EDM machined surface and compounds formed using Cu Ka radiation. Figure 2.7 presents the XRD

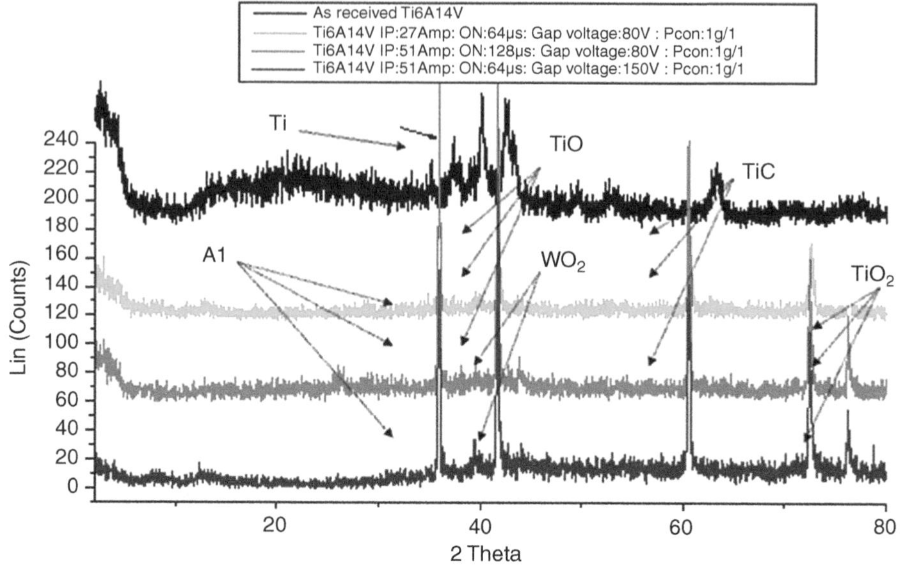

FIGURE 2.7 XRD pattern of nano aluminum PM-EDM on titanium alloy.

patterns of as received and nano aluminum PM-EDM on titanium alloy. It can be examined that most of the peaks match titanium peaks. The XRD pattern of machined titanium alloy by copper tungsten electrode indicates the formation of TiO_2, TiC, and WO2 including titanium phases as seen in Figure 2.7. Electric sparks generated during machining decompose the kerosene dielectric fluid into C and H and result in C deposited onto the machined surface. The transfer and deposit of alloying elements improve the machined surface properties particularly micro-hardness and fatigue.

2.8.10 Surface Sensitivity of Nano Aluminum PM-EDM on Titanium Alloy

X-ray photoelectron spectroscopy (XPS) techniques were used to analyze the chemical composition and oxidize amounts of the outermost machined surface and evaluate if there was any contamination from foreign particles. Figure 2.8 presents the XPS of the received titanium element and EDM machined surface PM-EDM, respectively. The XPS analysis shows changes in peak position and intensity of elements on the machined surfaces. Ti-6Al-4V alloy revealed the Ti_2p doublet peaks at 459.38eV and 465.8eV attributed to the Ti–Ti bond. Machined surfaces of EDM and PM-EDM on titanium alloy showed these peaks at slightly lower binding energies of 455.28 eV, which were attributed to Ti–O due to the release of oxygen during EDM and PM-EDM process. Titanium oxide layer forms on the titanium alloy implant surface protect the original metal from further oxidation and improves the osseointegration [63]. Ti-O is useful for the development of biocompatible coatings of human implants [64].

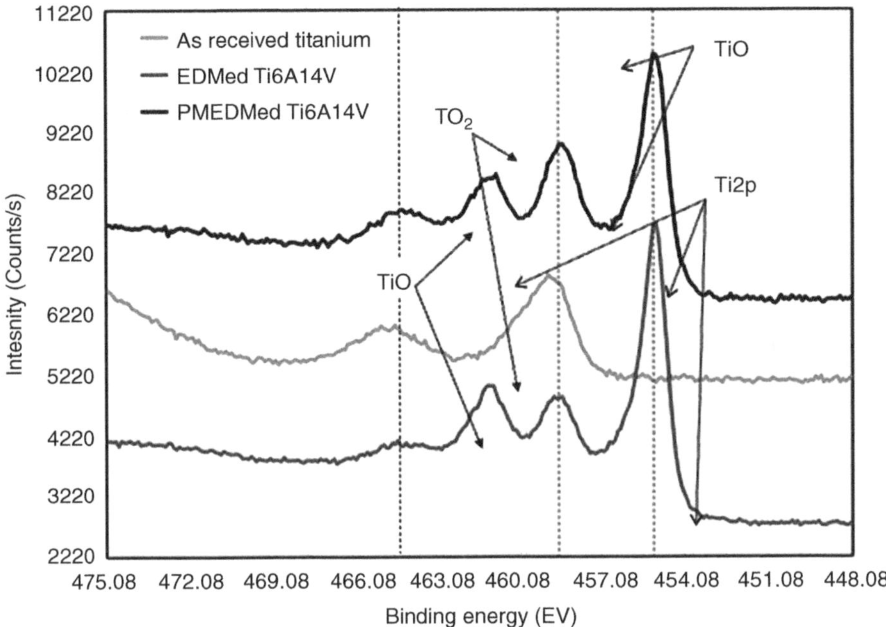

FIGURE 2.8 XPS of EDM (IP = 27 A, ON = 64 μs, GapV = 80 V and PM-EDM (IP = 27 A, ON = 64 μs, GapV = 80 V, Pcon = 1 g/l) on titanium alloy.

The binding energy for EDM and PM-EDM on titanium remains slightly the same for the various peaks.

The difference between EDM and PM-EDM on titanium alloy is that PM-EDM shows a pronounced intensity of photoelectron, and it measures how much of Ti_2p is at the surface. EDM and PM-EDM processes induce surface modification due to erosion of sparks. The presence of carbon is from EDM and PM-EDM processes which release carbon from the burning cycle. After XPS examinations of EDM and PM-EDM machined surfaces, the results of the titanium alloy machined surface show difference in term of machined surface compositions. For PM-EDM machine surface, the increase in the amount of nano aluminum and aluminum oxide by XPS measurements may be the proof of improvement of PM-EDM machined and responsible for corrosion resistance compared to conventional EDM.

2.8.11 Effects Plot for MRR on Nano Aluminum PM-EDM on Titanium Alloy

Figure 2.9 presents the plot of IP, ON-time, gap voltage, and nano aluminum concentration on MRR. More materials are removed from the workpiece with variation of IP, ON-time, and nano aluminum concentration. The improvement of MRR compared to conventional EDM on titanium alloy is due to accumulation of sparks between two consecutive nano aluminum particles in machining area results in series of discharges.

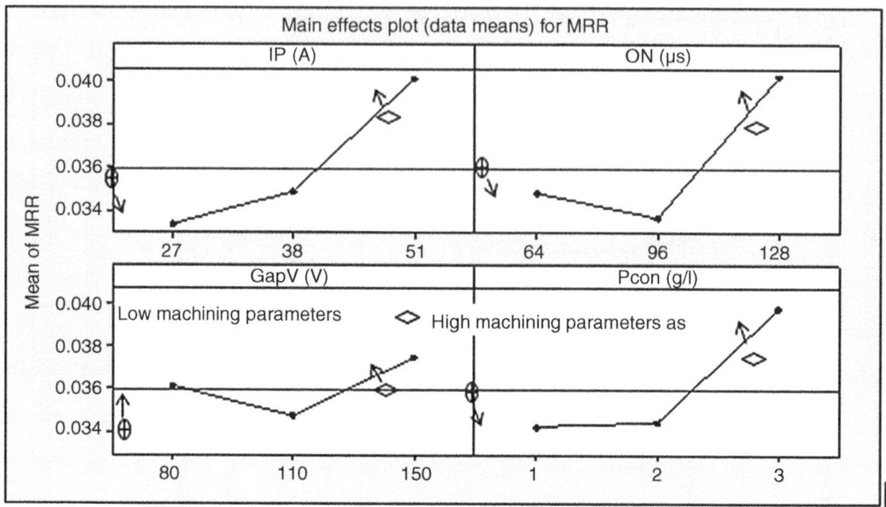

FIGURE 2.9 Effects plot for MRR (g/min) of nano aluminum PM-EDM on titanium alloy.

This increases the sparking intensity within discharges leading to faster erosion from the surface of the workpiece, and therefore increases MRR. MRR rapidly decreases with the variation of gap voltage from 80 to 110 V and this may be due to sparks formed between the electrode and workpiece obstructing the energy transfer, thus reducing MRR. It can conclude that the effect of parameters IP, ON-time, Pcon, and interaction GapV*Pcon on MRR is significant for nano aluminum PM-EDM on titanium alloy. With added nano aluminum, the MRR of nano aluminum PM-EDM is improved and about 40% increased as compared to MRR of conventional EDM on titanium alloy. The mathematical model for MRR of nano aluminum PM-EDM on titanium alloy and the considered process variables was obtained within 95% confidence interval after reducing the not significant terms as follows (Equation 2.4):

$$MRR = + 0.034 + 3.389E\text{-}003*A + 2.722E\text{-}003*B + 6.219E\text{-}004*C$$
$$+ 2.812E\text{-}003*D + 2.134E\text{-}003*C*D + 3.769E\text{-}003*B^2 \qquad (2.4)$$

where: A is the parameter IP; B, ON; C, gap voltage and D, powder concentration.

2.8.12 Interaction Plot for MRR of Nano Aluminum PM-EDM on Titanium Alloy

Figure 2.10 presents the interaction plot of machining parameters when machining titanium alloy using nano aluminum. It presents the interaction between four different machining parameters especially IP, ON, gap voltage, and nano aluminum concentration on MRR. This explains that the effect of one parameter is dependent upon another parameter, that is why there are no parallel trends in interaction plot. The spark energy increases with IP, ON-time, and gap voltage and hence, more MRR is achieved with IP, ON-time, and gap voltage.

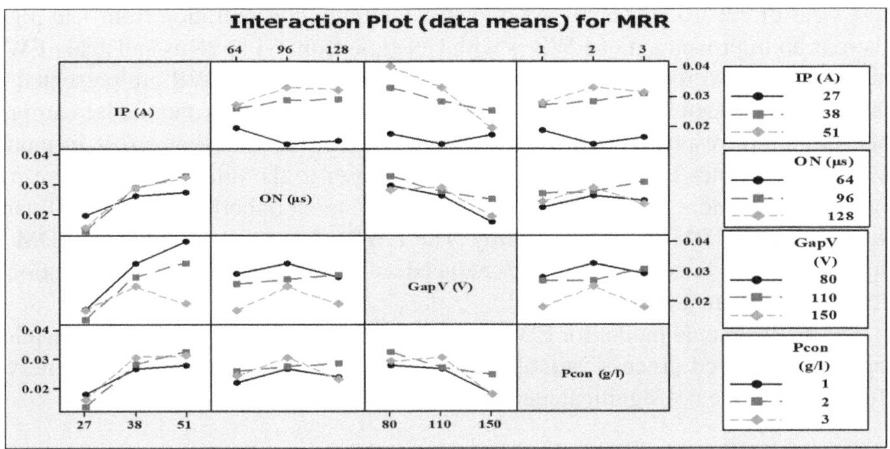

FIGURE 2.10 Interaction plot for MRR of nano aluminum PM-EDM on titanium alloy.

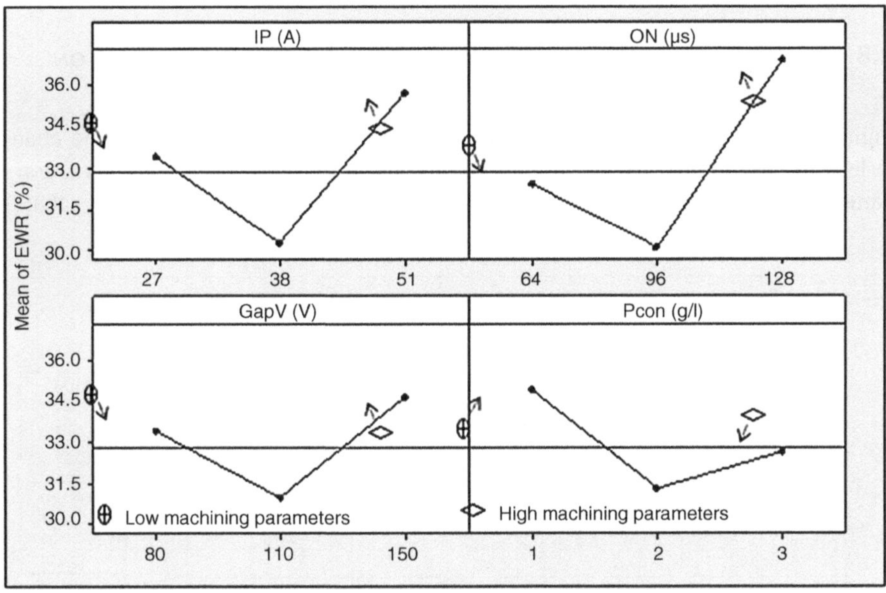

FIGURE 2.11 Effects plot for EWR of nano aluminum PM-EDM on titanium alloy.

2.8.13 EFFECTS PLOT FOR EWR OF NANO ALUMINUM PM-EDM ON TITANIUM ALLOY

Figure 2.11 presents the main effect of IP, ON-time, gap voltage, and nano aluminum concentration EWR when machining titanium alloy PM-EDM mixed dielectric fluid. Electrode slightly increases with variation of IP gap voltage from low values to the center point but rapidly increases with IP and gap voltage from center to high values.

Low wear of electrode is analyzed of nano aluminum concentration from 1 to 3 g/l. There is an improvement of EWR is with ON-time from 64 to 96 μs and again EWR increases from 96 to 128 μs. The regression coefficients for EWR are presented in Table A.4 in Appendix A with $R^2 = 72.6\%$. This indicates that the model can predict the output response with accuracy. The standard deviation of errors in model $S = 3.192$ indicates that the observed data are closer to the fitted line as Figure A.3 showed in Appendix A. Parameters ON-time is the most important for EWR of nano aluminum PM-EDM on titanium alloy. The EWR of nano aluminum PM-EDM is slightly improved and about 17.39% reduced as compared to EWR of conventional EDM on titanium alloy.

The mathematical model for EWR of nano aluminum PM-EDM on titanium alloy and the considered process variables was obtained within 95% confidence interval after reducing the not significant terms as follows (Equation 2.5):

$$EWR = +30.10 +2.28*B+4.59*B^2 \tag{2.5}$$

where: B is ON-time.

2.8.14 Interaction Plot for EWR of Nano Aluminum PM-EDM on Titanium Alloy

Figure 2.12 shows the interaction effects of machining parameters and the change in level of one or two parameters affect the output response. There is interaction of parameters on EWR at two different machining parameters and this indicates that the

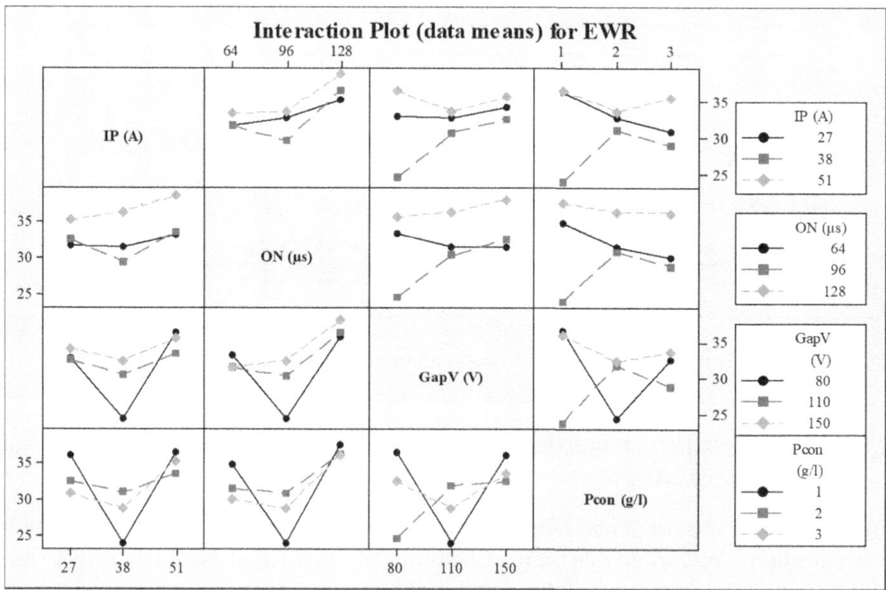

FIGURE 2.12 Interaction plot for EWR of nano aluminum PM-EDM on titanium alloy.

effect of one parameter is dependent upon another parameter because IP, ON-time, and gap voltage independently or combined control the discharge energy size. High set of IP, ON-time, or gap voltage increases the discharge energy.

2.8.15 Effects Plot for ROC of Nano Aluminum PM-EDM on Titanium Alloy

Figure 2.13 presents the main effect of IP, ON-time, gap voltage, and nano aluminum concentration on ROC. Overcut is getting wider when IP, ON-time, and gap voltage vary from low values to center point values and it is improved from center values to high values. The effect of nano aluminum concentration is more pronounced from 1 to 3 g/l. The mathematical model for ROC of nano aluminum PM-EDM on titanium alloy and the considered process variables was obtained within 95% confidence interval after reducing the not significant terms as follows (Equation 2.6):

$$ROC = +0.061 + 6.167E\text{-}003*A + 0.011*B \tag{2.6}$$

where: A is peak current and B, ON-time.

2.8.16 Regression Coefficients for Ra of Nano Aluminum PM-EDM on MHSS

Table 2.11 presents the estimated regression coefficients for surface roughness (Ra). It indicates that peak current has a significant effect on surface roughness followed by ON-time and interactions of ON*Pcon and GapV*Pcon.

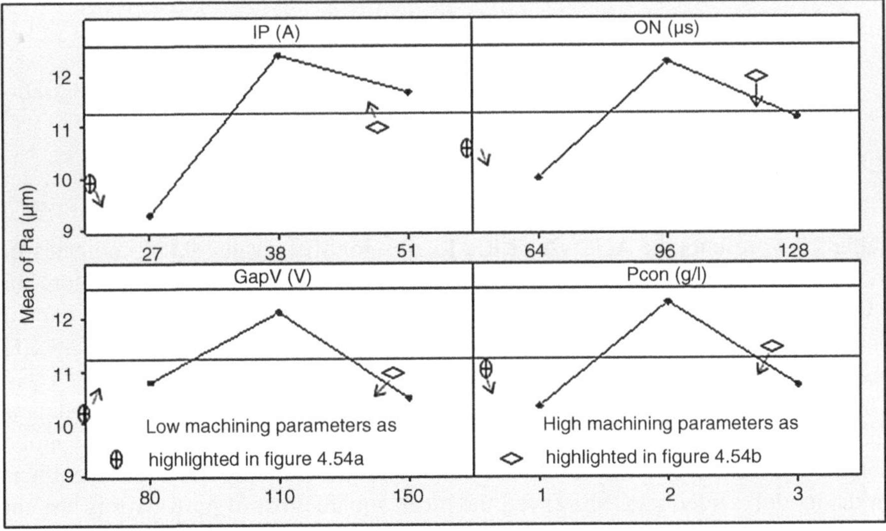

FIGURE 2.13   Effects plot for Ra of nano aluminum PM-EDM on MHSS.

TABLE 2.11
Regression coefficients for Ra of nano aluminum PM-EDM on MHSS

Term	Coef	SE Coef	*T*	*P*
Constant	12.6402	0.3617	34.950	0.000
IP	1.1947	0.2700	4.424	0.000
ON	0.5814	0.2700	2.153	0.048
GapV	-0.1577	0.2700	-0.584	0.568
Pcon	0.2142	0.2700	0.793	0.440
IP*IP	-1.3285	0.7170	-1.853	0.084
ON*ON	-0.3199	0.7116	-0.450	0.659
GapV*GapV	0.2101	0.7275	0.289	0.777
Pcon*Pcon	-0.8394	0.7116	-1.180	0.257
IP*ON	0.4196	0.2863	1.466	0.163
IP*GapV	-0.4456	0.2859	-1.558	0.140
IP*Pcon	0.4640	0.2863	1.621	0.126
ON*GapV	-0.2180	0.2860	-0.762	0.458
ON*Pcon	0.8178	0.2864	2.856	0.012
GapV*Pcon	0.7988	0.2860	2.792	0.014

$S = 1.145$ R-Sq = 82.7% R-Sq(adj) = 66.5%

The mathematical model for surface roughness of nano aluminum PM-EDM on molybdenum high-speed steel material and the considered process variables was obtained within 95% confidence interval after reducing the not significant terms as follows (Equation 2.7):

$$Ra = + 12.37 + 1.20*A + 0.58*B - 0.16*C + 0.21*D$$
$$+ 0.82*B*D + 0.80*C*D - 1.90*A{\wedge}2 \tag{2.7}$$

where: A is peak current; B, ON-time, C, gap voltage and D, powder concentration.

2.8.17 ANALYSIS OF VARIANCE FOR RA OF NANO ALUMINUM PM-EDM ON MHSS

Table 2.12 presents the ANOVA of Ra. Regression the *p*-value 0.002 indicates that the model is well fitted with lack-of-fit 6.99. The factors having *p*-value more than 0.05 are considered non-significant. The total error on regression is the sum of errors on linear, square, and interactions terms (93.969 = 31.083 + 31.728 + 31.158). The residual error is the sum of pure and lack-of-fit errors (19.682 = 18.368 + 1.314). The fit summary recommended that the linear, square, and interaction models are statistically significant for analysis of surface roughness of PM-EDM on molybdenum high steel, the *p*-value for the lack-of-fit is 0.022, which is not significant, so the model is adequate. Moreover, the mean square error of pure error is less than that of lack-of-fit.

TABLE 2.12
ANOVA for Ra of nano aluminum PM-EDM on MHSS

Source	df	Seq SS	Adj SS	Adj MS	F	P
Regression	14	93.969	93.969	6.7121	5.12	0.002
Linear	4	31.083	33.040	8.2600	6.30	0.004
Square	4	31.728	31.816	7.9540	6.06	0.004
Interaction	6	31.158	31.158	5.1930	3.96	0.014
Residual error	15	19.682	19.682	1.3121		
Lack-of-Fit	10	18.368	18.368	1.8368	6.99	0.022
Pure Error	5	1.314	1.314	0.2628		
Total	29	113.651				

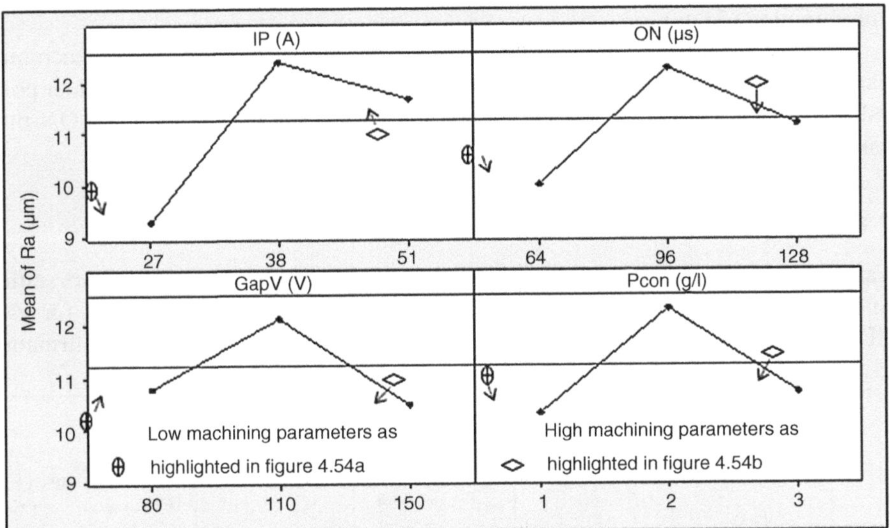

FIGURE 2.14   Effect plot for Ra of nano aluminum PM-EDM on MHSS.

2.8.18   EFFECTS PLOT FOR RA OF NANO ALUMINUM PM-EDM ON MHSS

Figure 2.14 presents the main effect of IP, ON-time, gap voltage, and nano aluminum concentration on Ra. Ra is getting rougher when any of the four machining parameters vary from low value to the center point value and then Ra decreases from the center point value to the high of each parameter. The increase in Ra to the optimum value is due to increased spark gap and instability of process. From the center point to the high setting for IP, ON-time, gap voltage, and powder concentration, the process is stable, and the electrical discharges are well distributed among the particles, which reduce the energy released from spark and reduced the surface roughness. Ra of PM-EDM on molybdenum high-speed steel is much improved as compared to Ra of EDM on molybdenum high-speed steel. Surface roughness of nano aluminum PM-EDM is slightly improved and about 16.21% reduced as compared to surface roughness of conventional EDM on molybdenum high-speed steel.

2.8.19 INTERACTION PLOT FOR Ra OF NANO ALUMINUM PM-EDM ON MHSS

Figure 2.15 presents the interaction effects of IP, ON-time, gap voltage, and nano aluminum concentration on MRR and the change in level of one or two machining parameters affect the output response. There is an interaction between any two machining parameters combinations because discharge spark energy is function of IP, ON-time, and gap voltage. Figure 2.16 presents response surface for Ra subjected to the machining parameters of IP and ON-time, while gap voltage and nano aluminum concentration remain constant at the center point value. It can be analyzed that Ra tends to increase with the increase in IP for any value of ON-time and inversely. Minimum Ra value of around 7 μm is obtained at low peak current (27 A) and low pulse on time (64 μs).

Figure 2.17 presents 3D surface response for Ra in relation to the machining parameters of IP and ON-time, while gap voltage remains constant at the center point values. The increase in surface roughness with increasing peak current and ON-time can be analyzed.

2.8.20 VALIDATION TEST

Validation tests were run with some selected predicted machining parameters setting to test at the optimal factor's levels. Table 2.13 presents the volition test for PM-EDM on titanium alloy, Table 2.14 for EDM on titanium alloy. Five confirmation

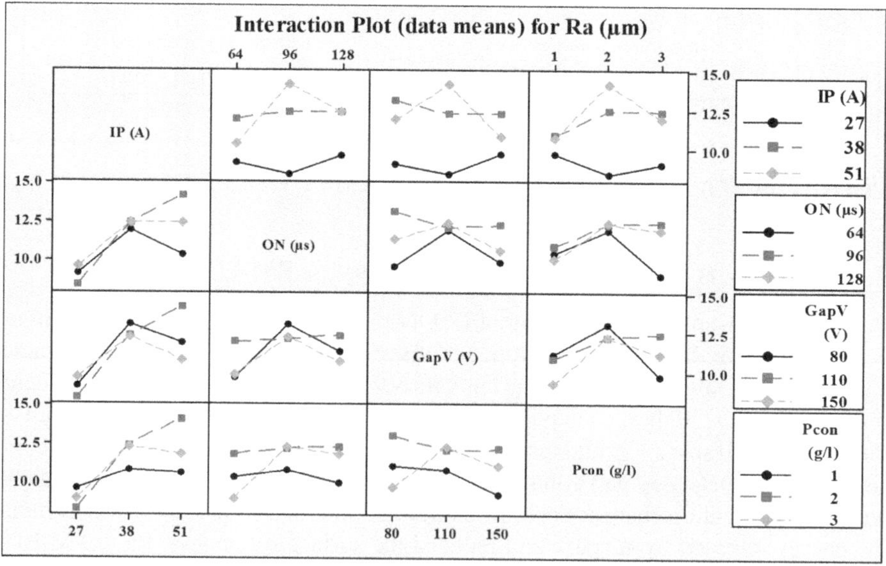

FIGURE 2.15   Interaction plot for Ra of nano aluminum PM-EDM on MHSS.

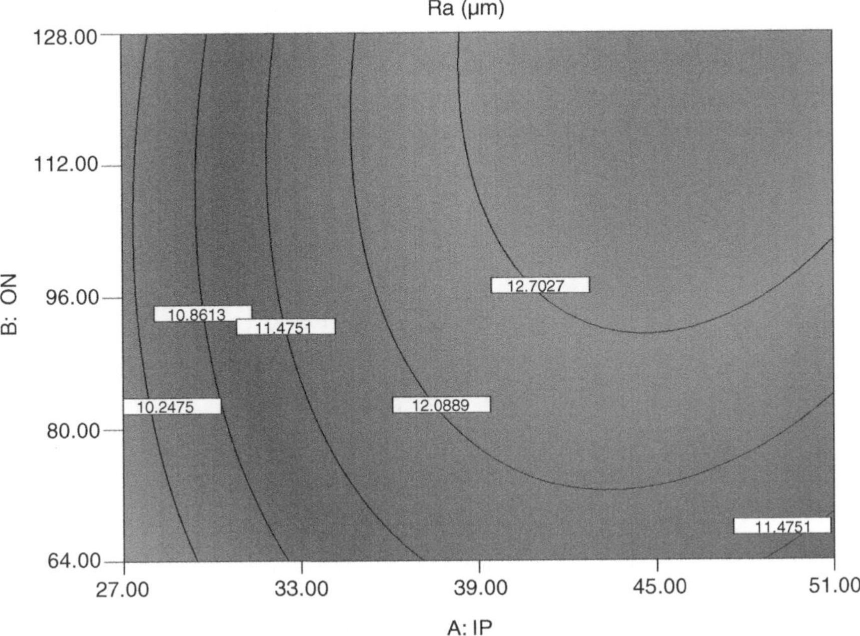

FIGURE 2.16 Contour plot for machined surface roughness of nano aluminum PM-EDM on MHSS.

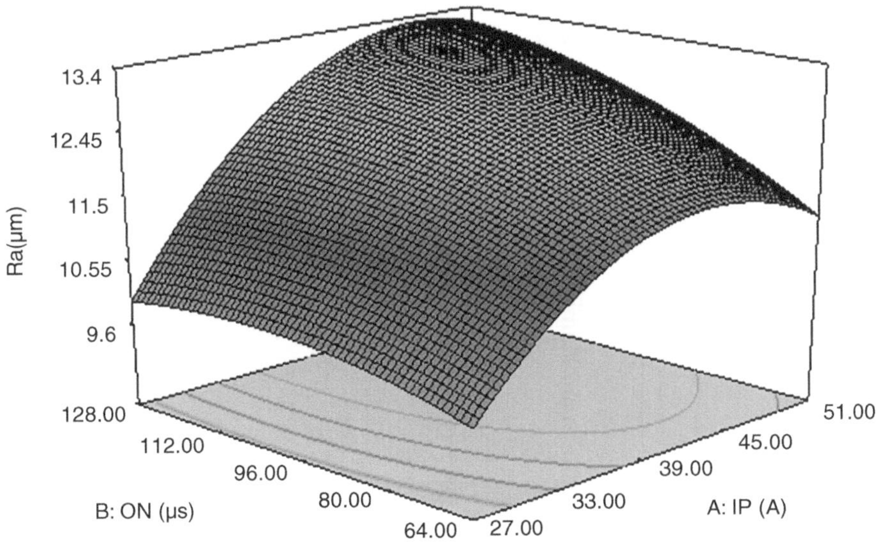

FIGURE 2.17 Plot depicting machined surface roughness of nano aluminum PM-EDM on MHSS.

TABLE 2.13
Validation test for nano aluminum PM-EDM on titanium alloy

No	IP	ON	GapV	Pcon	Ra			MRR			EWR			ROC		
					Pred	Actual	Error (%)	Pred	Actual	Error (%)	Pred	Actual	Error (%)	Pred	Actual	Error (%)
1	37.85	64	80	3	7.501	7.825	4.13	0.037	0.041	9.80	13.53	12.751	-6.08	0.056	0.059	4.87
11	40.41	64	81.32	3	7.749	7.315	-5.93	0.039	0.043	8.36	14.10	13.537	-4.15	0.059	0.061	4.68
13	31.79	64	80	3	7.298	6.778	-7.68	0.030	0.027	-9.03	13.19	12.875	-2.43	0.049	0.055	9.47
16	35.36	64	80	1	6.082	6.473	6.05	0.032	0.029	-10.54	20.71	18.752	-10.43	0.055	0.063	12.36
23	34.28	128	89.75	1	7.275	7.564	3.83	0.030	0.028	-7.59	23.53	22.465	-4.72	0.072	0.065	-10.48

TABLE 2.14
Validation test for nano aluminum PM-EDM on MHSS

No	IP	ON	Gap	Pcon	Ra			MRR			EWR			ROC		
					Pred	Actual	Error (%)	Pred	Actual	Error (%)	Pred	Actual	Error (%)	Pred	Actual	Error (%)
1	50.23	64	146.88	1	9.743	10.253	4.97	0.533	0.601	11.30	1.534	1.445	-6.14	0.092	0.101	9.62
2	46.61	64	149.98	1.01	10.320	9.717	-6.21	0.511	0.474	-7.85	1.522	1.486	-2.41	0.084	0.092	8.64
3	42.95	64	150	1.01	10.712	11.645	8.01	0.484	0.435	-11.21	1.582	1.722	8.15	0.075	0.081	8.07
5	30.5	128	150	1	8.858	9.632	8.03	0.393	0.4313	8.96	1.429	1.532	6.74	0.087	0.081	-7.74
7	27	128	140.59	1	8.147	7.356	-10.75	0.350	0.382	8.41	1.593	1.461	-9.01	0.083	0.076	-8.12

experiments have been conducted at the optimum settings of the process parameters. Analyses of the validation experiments show that the actual values of Ra, MRR, TWR, and OC are within 95% of the prediction interval. Due to error percentage which is, in all most cases less than 10%, it can conclude that indicates that the empirical models developed in this work are reasonably reliable for prediction of Ra, MRR, TWR, and OC with a respective acceptable error.

2.9 CONCLUSIONS

In this research, it is established that the use of PM-EDM improves the surface quality on titanium alloy for biomedical and industrial applications. PM-EDM reduces the surface roughness, micro-cracks, craters, and voids on the machined surface. This is attributed due to transfer of alloying elements deposited and uniform distribution of particles from nano aluminum onto the machined surface. The created carbon enriched surface layer also improves osseointegration of the titanium alloy workpiece.

Experiments were run using a designed and fabricated PM-EDM open system.

1. The new PM-EDM open system was successfully designed, fabricated, tested, and analyzed.
2. Ra, MRR, EWR, and ROC of nano aluminum PM-EDM on titanium are, respectively, 38.46% reduced, 40% increased, 17.39% reduced, and 16.66% reduced as compared to Ra, MRR, EWR, and ROC of conventional EDM on titanium alloy.
3. Ra, MRR, EWR, and ROC of nano aluminum PM-EDM on molybdenum high-speed steel are, respectively, 16.21% reduced, 17.5% increased, 37.77% reduced, and 16.66% reduced as compared to Ra, MRR, EWR, and ROC of conventional EDM.
4. Nano tungsten PM-EDM on molybdenum high-speed steel is slightly improved with Ra which is about 10.8% reduced; EWR and ROC are reduced about 16.66% and 9.1%, respectively, as compared to conventional EDM on molybdenum high-speed steel.
5. Tungsten PM-EDM with surfactant of molybdenum high-speed steel is not much improved as compared to EDM and PM-EDM of molybdenum high-speed steel.
6. The use of nano aluminum in PM-EDM on titanium alloy and molybdenum high-speed steel results in good output results as compared to nano tungsten powder PM-EDM.
7. PM-EDM marginally enhanced corrosion rate on titanium alloy due to the deposited and embedment of nano aluminum on machined surface. Corrosion is 41.97% reduced when using aluminum PM-EDM on titanium alloy as compared to corrosion of conventional EDM on titanium alloy. PM-EDM is explored to have potential in biomedical and industry applications.
8. Generate the mathematical models and statistical analysis of output responses namely surface roughness, MRR, EWR subjected to EDM input machining parameters.
9. Synthesize the optimal PM-EDM and EDM parameters on titanium alloy and molybdenum high-speed steel tool using nano aluminum and nano tungsten.

REFERENCES

[1] K. Ho and S. Newman, "State of the art electrical discharge machining (EDM)," *International Journal of Machine Tools and Manufacture*, vol. 43, pp. 1287–1300, 2003.

[2] M. Kunleda, Y. Miyoshi, T. Takaya, N. Nakajima, Y. ZhanBo, and M. Yoshida, "High speed 3D milling by dry EDM," *CIRP Annals-Manufacturing Technology*, vol. 52, pp. 147–150, 2003.

[3] P. Sreejith and B. Ngoi, "Dry machining: machining of the future," *Journal of Materials Processing Technology*, vol. 101, pp. 287–291, 2000.

[4] C. Kao, J. Tao, and A. J. Shih, "Near dry electrical discharge machining," *International Journal of Machine Tools and Manufacture*, vol. 47, pp. 2273–2281, 2007.

[5] Z. Yu, T. Jun, and K. Masanori, "Dry electrical discharge machining of cemented carbide," *Journal of Materials Processing Technology*, vol. 149, pp. 353–357, 2004.

[6] J. Tao, "Investigation of dry and near-dry electrical discharge milling processes," phd, Mechanical engineering, University of Michigan, Michigan, 2008.

[7] A. Gholipoor, H. Baseri, and M. R. Shabgard, "Investigation of near dry EDM compared with wet and dry EDM processes," *Journal of Mechanical Science and Technology*, vol. 29, pp. 2213–2218, 2015.

[8] L. Liqing and S. Yingjie, "Study of dry EDM with oxygen-mixed and cryogenic cooling approaches," *Procedia CIRP*, vol. 6, pp. 344–350, 2013.

[9] Q. Zhang, J. Zhang, J. Deng, Y. Qin, and Z. Niu, "Ultrasonic vibration electrical discharge machining in gas," *Journal of Materials Processing Technology*, vol. 129, pp. 135–138, 2002.

[10] Q. Zhang, R. Du, J. Zhang, and Q. Zhang, "An investigation of ultrasonic-assisted electrical discharge machining in gas," *International Journal of Machine Tools and Manufacture*, vol. 46, pp. 1582–1588, 2006.

[11] Q. Zhang, J. Zhang, S. Ren, J. Deng, and X. Ai, "Study on technology of ultrasonic vibration aided electrical discharge machining in gas," *Journal of Materials Processing Technology*, vol. 149, pp. 640–644, 2004.

[12] A. Abdullah and M. R. Shabgard, "Effect of ultrasonic vibration of tool on electrical discharge machining of cemented tungsten carbide (WC-Co)," *The International Journal of Advanced Manufacturing Technology*, vol. 38, pp. 1137–1147, 2008.

[13] C. Praneetpongrung, Y. Fukuzawa, S. Nagasawa, and K. Yamashita, "Effects of the EDM combined ultrasonic vibration on the machining properties of Si3N4," *Materials Transactions*, vol. 51, p. 2113, 2010.

[14] J. Sing, R. Walia, P. Satsangi, and V. Singh, "Hybrid electric discharge machining process with continuous and discontinuous ultrasonic vibrations on workpiece," *International Journal of Mechanic Systems Engineering*, vol. 2, 2012.

[15] T. T. Endo, Takayuki. Mitsui, Kimiyuki, "Study of vibration-assisted micro-EDM--The effect of vibration on machining time and stability of discharge," *Precision Engineering*, vol. 32, pp. 269–277, 2008.

[16] S. Singh and A. Pandey, "Some Studies into electrical dDischarge machining of nimonic75 super alloy using rotary copper disk electrode," *Journal of Materials Engineering and Performance*, vol. 22, pp. 1290–1303, 2013.

[17] H.-M. Chow, L.-D. Yang, C.-T. Lin, and Y.-F. Chen, "The use of SiC powder in water as dielectric for micro-slit EDM machining," *Journal of Materials Processing Technology*, vol. 195, pp. 160–170, 2008.

[18] H. Chow, B. Yan, and F. Huang, "Micro slit machining using electro-discharge machining with a modified rotary disk electrode (RDE)," *Journal of Materials Processing Technology*, vol. 91, pp. 161–166, 1999.

[19] K. Chattopadhyay, S. Verma, P. Satsangi, and P. Sharma, "Development of empirical model for different process parameters during rotary electrical discharge machining of copper–steel (EN-8) system," *Journal of Materials Processing Technology*, vol. 209, pp. 1454–1465, 2009.

[20] Y.-C. C. Lin, Yuan-Feng. Wang, Der-An. Lee, Ho-Shiun, "Optimization of machining parameters in magnetic force assisted EDM based on Taguchi method," *Journal of Materials Processing Technology*, vol. 209, pp. 3374–3383, 2009.

[21] Y. Liu, C. Wang, Y. Zhang, S. Xiao, and Y. Chen, "Fractal process and particle size distribution in a TiH 2 powder milling system," *Powder Technology*, vol. 284, pp. 272–278, 2015.

[22] W. Zhao, Q. Meng, and Z. Wang, "The application of research on powder mixed EDM in rough machining," *Journal of Materials Processing Technology*, vol. 129, pp. 30–33, 2002.

[23] S. Singh, S. Maheshwari, A. Dey, and P. Pandey, "Experimental results and analysis for Electrical Discharge Machining (EDM) of aluminium metal matrix composites with powder-mixed dielectric: Lenth's method," *International Journal of Manufacturing Technology and Management*, vol. 21, pp. 67–82, 2010.

[24] B. Özerkan and C. Çoğun, "Effect of powder mixed dielectric on machining performance in electric discharge machining (EDM)," *Gazi University Journal of Science*, vol. 18, pp. 211–228, 2010.

[25] B. Singh, J. Kumar, and S. Kumar, "Investigation of the rool wear rate in tungsten powder-mixed electric discharge machining of AA6061/10% SiCp composite," *Materials and Manufacturing Processes*, vol. 31, pp. 456–466, 2016.

[26] B. Kuriachen and J. Mathew, "Effect of Powder mixed mielectric on material removal and surface modification in microelectric discharge machining of Ti-6Al-4V," *Materials and Manufacturing Processes*, vol. 31, pp. 439–446, 2016.

[27] S. Singh, S. Maheshwari, and P. Pandey, "An experimental investigation into abrasive electrical discharge machining (AEDM) of Al_2O_3 particulate reinforced Al-based metal matrix composites," *Journal of Mechanical Engineering*, vol. 7, pp. 13–33, 2006.

[28] J. Kozak and K. Rajurkar, "Hybrid machining process evaluation and development," in *Proceedings of the 2th Intern. Conference on Machining and Measurements of Sculptured Surfaces. Krakow*, 2000, pp. 501–536.

[29] Y. Uno, A. Okada, and S. Cetin, "Surface modification of EDMed surface with powder mixed fluid," in *2nd International Conference on Design and Production of Dies and Molds, Kuşadası*, 2001.

[30] H. M. Chow, B. H. Yan, F. Y. Huang, and J. C. Hung, "Study of added powder in kerosene for the micro-slit machining of titanium alloy using electro-discharge machining," *Journal of Materials Processing Technology*, vol. 101, pp. 95–103, 2000.

[31] P. Pecas and E. Henriques, "Electrical discharge machining using simple and powder-mixed dielectric: The effect of the electrode area in the surface roughness and topography," *Journal of Materials Processing Technology*, vol. 200, pp. 250–258, 2008.

[32] S. Padhee, N. Nayak, S. Panda, P. Dhal, and S. Mahapatra, "Multi-objective parametric optimization of powder mixed electro-discharge machining using response surface methodology and non-dominated sorting genetic algorithm," *Sadhana*, vol. 37, pp. 223–240, 2012.

[33] S. Kumar and U. Batra, "Surface modification of die steel materials by EDM method using tungsten powder-mixed dielectric," *Journal of Manufacturing Processes*, vol. 14, pp. 35–40, 2012.

[34] H. Kansal, S. Singh, and P. Kumar, "Parametric optimization of powder mixed electrical discharge machining by response surface methodology," *Journal of Materials Processing Technology*, vol. 169, pp. 427–436, 2005.

[35] H. Kansal, S. Singh, and P. Kumar, "Effect of silicon powder mixed EDM on machining rate of AISI D2 die steel," *Journal of Manufacturing Processes*, vol. 9, pp. 13–22, 2007.

[36] P. Peças and E. Henriques, "Effect of the powder concentration and dielectric flow in the surface morphology in electrical discharge machining with powder-mixed dielectric (PMD-EDM)," *The International Journal of Advanced Manufacturing Technology*, vol. 37, pp. 1120–1132, 2008.

[37] S. Singh, H. Singh, J. Singh, and R. Bhatiac, "Effect of composition of powder mixed dielectric fluid on performance of electric discharge machining," *Materials Science and Engineering*, vol. 2, 2011.

[38] K. Ojha, R. Garg, and K. Singh, "Experimental Investigation and modeling of PMEDM process with chromium powder suspended dielectric," *International Journal of Applied Science and Engineering*, vol. 9, pp. 65–81, 2011.

[39] A. S. Gill and S. Kumar, "Surface alloying of H11 die steel by tungsten using EDM process," *The International Journal of Advanced Manufacturing Technology*, pp. 1–9, 2015.

[40] J. Stráský, J. Havlíková, L. Bačáková, P. Harcuba, M. Mhaede, and M. Janeček, "Characterization of electric discharge machining, subsequent etching and shot-peening as a surface treatment for orthopedic implants," *Applied Surface Science*, vol. 281, pp. 73–78, 2013.

[41] M. Kunieda, M. Yoshida, and N. Taniguchi, "Electrical discharge machining in gas," *CIRP Annals-Manufacturing Technology*, vol. 46, pp. 143–146, 1997.

[42] P. Singh, A. Kumar, N. Beri, and V. Kumar, "Influence of electrical parameters in powder mixed elecric discharge machining (PMEDM) of hastelloy," *Journal of Engineering Research and Studies E-ISSN*, vol. 976, p. 7916, 2010.

[43] M. Rajendra and G. Rao, "Experimental evaluation of performance of electrical discharge machining of D3 die steel with Al2O3 abrasive mixed dielectric material by using design of experiments," *International Journal of Scientific Engineering and Technology*, vol. 3, pp. 599–606, 2014.

[44] S. Singh and M.-F. Yeh, "Optimization of abrasive powder mixed EDM of aluminum matrix composites with multiple responses using gray relational analysis," *Journal of Materials Engineering and Performance*, vol. 21, pp. 481–491, 2012.

[45] A. Batish and A. Bhattacharya, "Mechanism of material deposition from powder, electrode and dielectric for surface modification of H11 and H13 die steels in EDM process," *Materials Science Forum*, 2012, pp. 61–75.

[46] F. Q. Hu, B. Y. Song, Y. Guo, X. Yang, J. Bai, and D. Li, "Study on powder mixed EDM of an aluminium matrix composite," *Advanced Materials Research*, vol. 183, pp. 1947–1951, 2011.

[47] Y.-F. Tzeng and C.-Y. Lee, "Effects of powder characteristics on electrodischarge machining efficiency," *The International Journal of advanced manufacturing technology*, vol. 17, pp. 586–592, 2001.

[48] Y.-f. Tzeng and F.-c. Chen, "Multi-objective optimisation of high-speed electrical discharge machining process using a Taguchi fuzzy-based approach," *Materials & Design*, vol. 28, pp. 1159–1168, 2007.

[49] Y. Wong, L. Lim, I. Rahuman, and W. Tee, "Near-mirror-finish phenomenon in EDM using powder-mixed dielectric," *Journal of Materials Processing Technology*, vol. 79, pp. 30–40, 1998.

[50] C. Cogun, B. Özerkan, and T. Karacay, "An experimental investigation on the effect of powder mixed dielectric on machining performance in electric discharge machining," *Proceedings of the Institution of Mechanical Engineers, Part B: Journal of Engineering Manufacture*, vol. 220, pp. 1035–1050, 2006.

[51] J. Strasky, M. Janecek, and P. Harcuba, "Electric discharge machining of Ti-6Al-4V alloy for biomedical use," in *WDS*, pp. 127–131.

[52] C. Croarkin and P. Tobias, "*NIST/SEMATECH e-handbook of statistical methods*," NIST/SEMATECH, July. Available online: www.itl.nist.gov/div898/handbook, 2006.

[53] A. Standard, "B46. 1-2002," *Surface texture (Surface roughness, waviness, and lay)*, The American Society of Mechanical Engineers, An American National Standard, New York, pp. 1–98, 2002.

[54] R. DAS, M. Pradhan, and C. Das, "Prediction of surface roughness in electrical discharge machining of SKD 11 tool steel using recurrent Elman Networks," *JJMIE*, vol. 7, 2013.

[55] P. Harcuba, L. Bačáková, J. Stráský, M. Bačáková, K. Novotná, and M. Janeček, "Surface treatment by electric discharge machining of Ti–6Al–4V alloy for potential application in orthopaedics," *Journal of the Mechanical Behavior of Biomedical Materials*, vol. 7, pp. 96–105, 2012.

[56] E. Astm, "384." Standard test method for microhardness of materials," *American Society for Testing and Materials ASTM, Annual Book of Standards*, vol. 3, 1999.

[57] L. Tarasov and N. Thibault, "Determination of Knoop hardness numbers independent of load," *Transactions ASM*, vol. 38, pp. 331–353, 1947.

[58] H. Sidhom, F. Ghanem, T. Amadou, G. Gonzalez, and C. Braham, "Effect of electro discharge machining (EDM) on the AISI316L SS white layer microstructure and corrosion resistance," *The International Journal of Advanced Manufacturing Technology*, vol. 65, pp. 141–153, 2013.

[59] A. Casagrande, G. Cammarota, and L. Micele, "Relationship between fatigue limit and Vickers hardness in steels," *Materials Science and Engineering: A*, vol. 528, pp. 3468–3473, 2011.

[60] H. R. A. Bidhendi and M. Pouranvari, "Corrosion study of metallic biomaterials in simulated body fluid," *Metalurgija-M J o M*, vol. 17, pp. 13–22, 2011.

[61] N. Zaveri, G. D. McEwen, R. Karpagavalli, and A. Zhou, "Biocorrosion studies of TiO2 nanoparticle-coated Ti–6Al–4V implant in simulated biofluids," *Journal of Nanoparticle Research*, vol. 12, pp. 1609–1623, 2010.

[62] M. Mohanty, S. Baby, and K. Menon, "Spinal fixation device: a 6-year postimplantation study," *Journal of Biomaterials Applications*, vol. 18, pp. 109–121, 2003.

[63] G. A. Castilho, M. D. Martins, and W. A. Macedo, "Surface characterization of titanium based dental implants," *Brazilian Journal of Physics*, vol. 36, pp. 1004–1008, 2006.

[64] Z. Li, Y. Wu, and S. Miyake, "Metallic sputtering growth of high quality anatase phase TiO 2 films by inductively coupled plasma assisted DC reactive magnetron sputtering," *Surface and Coatings Technology*, vol. 203, pp. 3661–3668, 2009

3 Surface Analysis of Magnesium Alloy Processed Using C-EDM and PM-EDM Method

Muhammad Al'Hapis Abdul Razak, Ahmad Majdi Abdul-Rani, Iqtidar Ahmed Gul, Elhuseini Garba, Syed Shehzeb Abdullah, and Anas Ahmed

3.1 INTRODUCTION

Magnesium alloy has the potential to be applied in temporary orthopedic implants [1, 2]. However, magnesium alloy is considered as difficult-to-machine material due to low melting point which is 650°C, and this metal is only stable below its melting point [3]. Dull tool edge can lead to bad accuracy, excess heat, and spark to ignite at the edge of cutting tool. It is vital to avoid emulsion type coolant and water due to risk of fire hazard [4]. The spark erosion process is an alternative machining method normally applied on a challenging workpiece with intricate details. This machining method is categorized as one of thermal energy processes (TEPs) because the metal removal occurs due to high temperature and the most commonly used TEP is electro-discharge machining (EDM).

Conventional EDM (C-EDM) suffers of inconsistent machined surface quality and the formation of micro-cracks and craters on the machined surface. Furthermore, the application of electric current changes the mechanical properties of the machined surface [5]. In recent years, new exploratory research works have been initiated to improve the efficiency of EDM process using powder mixed EDM (PM-EDM) method [3, 6]. The PM-EDM method may lead to improve machined part surface finish [7]. The objective of this chapter is to analyze the surface quality of magnesium alloy processed using C-EDM and PM-EDM method. It is hypothesized that the surface quality of magnesium alloy processed using PM-EDM method will be smoother than C-EDM method.

3.2 LITERATURE REVIEW

Machining hard metals become easier using EDM process. Regardless of their hardness and strength, any electrically conductive metals can be machined by EDM

DOI: 10.1201/9781003456018-3

[8]. With EDM process, machining accuracy as small as 1 μm can be achieved. An exact shape as the electrode will be obtained on the specimen even though the shape is complex and designed with tight tolerance. The EDM operation inputs and programming are easier to be done using computerized machining control system. Unlike the traditional machining, during EDM process, there is no contact between the electrode and specimen making it a totally stress-free machining. Last but not least, the machined surface is also free from burrs.

The application of EDM process is only to machine the conductive materials [9]. Even though recently, there are works done by researchers to machine non-conductive materials using EDM by applying assisting electrode on top of the material surface [10], it is still under research and inconclusive. Compared to the traditional machining such as milling and turning, the cost of EDM process is comparatively more expensive. The electrode used in the process will be wearing and the machining time can be long depending on the operation inputs. There are also very limited references on the operation inputs available. Normally, machine user manual is only providing operation inputs to process steel-based metal and aluminum. Therefore, there is still a wide range of research can be conducted related to the EDM process.

During PM-EDM process, the powder suspended in the dielectric fluid reduces the insulating strength of dielectric fluid, reduce the energy density on the workpiece and increases the spark gap distance between the workpiece and tool-electrode. Thus, the plasma channel will enlarge and widen. With optimum powder concentration, the process become more stable with higher spark frequency generated and ensures a homogeneous distribution of the discharge energy which creating uniform erosion from the workpiece and results in shallow craters that served to improve the surface finish [11–14].

3.3 EXPERIMENTAL PROCEDURES

The data collected from C-EDM and PM-EDM experiments presented in this chapter were quantitative and used to describe the relationship among the operation inputs. Taguchi method was applied in designing the experiments and analyzing the results due to the suitability of the method to achieve research objectives. The orthogonal array was designed with three levels and four factors. In C-EDM experiments, the factors involve peak current (38, 47, and 55 A), gap voltage (80, 220, and 320 V), pulse on-time (16, 32, and 64 μs), and pulse off-time (128, 256, and 512 μs) as shown in Table 3.1. The lowest, medium, and highest notches were applied in the experiment. In PM-EDM experiments, the factors involve zinc powder concentration (1, 2, and 3 g/l), peak current (38, 47, and 55 A), pulse on-time (16, 32, and 64 μs), and pulse off-time (128, 256, and 512 μs) as shown in Table 3.2. The gap voltage as found less significant in C-EDM experiments was remained constant at the optimal value, 80 V in PM-EDM experiments.

The main facilities used for testing and analysis in this research were surface roughness tester and scanning electron microscopy (SEM) with energy-dispersive X-ray (EDX) spectroscope (SEM/EDS). Mitutoyo SurfTest SV-3000 with Mitutoyo SURFPAK-SV Version 1.201 surface roughness tester was used in this research to

TABLE 3.1
C-EDM experiment levels and factors

Factor	Level 1	Level 2	Level 3
Peak current (A)	38 A	47 A	55 A
Voltage (V)	80 V	220 V	320 V
Pulse on-time (μs)	16 μs	32 μs	64 μs
Pulse off-time (μs)	128 μs	256 μs	512 μs

TABLE 3.2
PM-EDM experiment levels and factors

Factor	Level 1	Level 2	Level 3
Powder concentration (g/l)	1 g/l	2 g/l	3g/l
Peak current (A)	38 A	47 A	55 A
Pulse on-time (μs)	16 μs	32 μs	64 μs
Pulse off-time (μs)	128 μs	256 μs	512 μs

analyze the roughness of affected magnesium alloy surfaces after being processed by C-EDM and PM-EDM method. Phenom ProX desktop type SEM/EDS was used to capture the machined surface images for morphological analysis purposes and analyzing the composed elements at a specific location on the machined surface.

3.4 RESULTS AND DISCUSSION

3.4.1 SURFACE ANALYSIS OF C-EDM EXPERIMENTS

An initiative has been taken to analyzing and synthesizing the effects of C-EDM operation inputs on the magnesium alloy machined surface. Before the experiments were conducted, it was hypothesized that the combination of lower peak current, lower gap voltage, lower pulse on-time, and higher pulse off-time would obtain the lower surface roughness. The smoother magnesium alloy machined surface was expected to result in a lower corrosion rate and the rougher magnesium alloy machined surface was expected to result in higher corrosion rate because the smoother machined surface will have smaller exposed surface area to contact with the solution during the corrosion test and the rougher machined surface will have larger exposed surface area to contact with the solution during the corrosion test [2]. The C-EDM experiments were conducted with three levels and four operation inputs. There were three times of replication for each combination. The data collected from three replicated experiments are presented in Table 3.3. The average surface roughness of all three replications is indicated in the right column. The early assumption that can be made based on the direct data was that the experiment 8 (processed with 55 A peak current, 220 V gap

TABLE 3.3
Surface roughness of C-EDM experiments

| | Controlled operation inputs | | | | Surface roughness (µm) | | | |
Exp.	Peak current (A)	Gap voltage (V)	Pulse on-time (µs)	Pulse off-time (µs)	Specimen 1	Specimen 2	Specimen 3	Average
1	38	80	16	128	6.889	6.393	6.237	6.506
2	38	220	32	256	8.313	8.390	8.199	8.301
3	38	320	64	512	11.872	11.654	12.887	12.138
4	47	80	32	512	6.661	7.999	6.739	7.133
5	47	220	64	128	12.766	12.412	14.404	13.194
6	47	320	16	256	5.997	6.033	6.942	6.324
7	55	80	64	256	12.327	13.356	13.764	13.149
8	55	220	16	512	5.366	6.227	6.186	5.926
9	55	320	32	128	9.228	8.310	8.725	8.754

voltage, 16 µs pulse on-time, and 512 µs pulse off-time) obtained the lowest surface roughness value with 5.926 µm. On the other hand, experiment 5 (processed with 47 A peak current, 220 V gap voltage, 64 µs pulse on-time, and 128 µs pulse off-time) obtained the highest surface roughness value with 13.149 µm.

From the collected data as presented in Table 3.3, it was found that the experiments 3, 5, and 7 which were conducted using the highest pulse on-time (64 µs) obtained the higher surface roughness values (>12 µm) and the experiments 1, 6, and 8 which utilized the lowest pulse on-time (16 µs) obtained the lower surface roughness values (<7 µm). Meanwhile, the experiments 2, 4, and 9 which were conducted using the medium pulse on-time (32 µs) obtained comparatively medium surface roughness values (7–9 µm). It can be presumed that the pulse on-time was directly proportional to the response. On the other hand, the other three operation inputs were not directly or inversely proportional to the surface roughness. For instance, even though there were three experiments conducted using the same peak current, the results varied. The same situation happened to the gap voltage and pulse on-time. However, all these assumptions were definitely not an accurate conclusion because they were only based on the collected data and yet to be analyzed thoroughly.

3.4.1.1 Main Effects Plot on the Surface Roughness of C-EDM Experiments

The data were then further analyzed to rank the operation inputs from the most significant to least significant affecting the surface roughness. The main effects plot of data means will reveal the exact combination of the operation inputs to obtain the lowest and the highest surface roughness within the examined limits. Figure 3.1 presents the main effects plot of data means, together with the value of the response of means. The lowest response values of each operation input can be found from the points A2, B1, C1, and D3 with the response values of 8.884, 8.929, 6.252, and 8.399 µm, respectively. In different words, the combination of operation inputs value of A2,

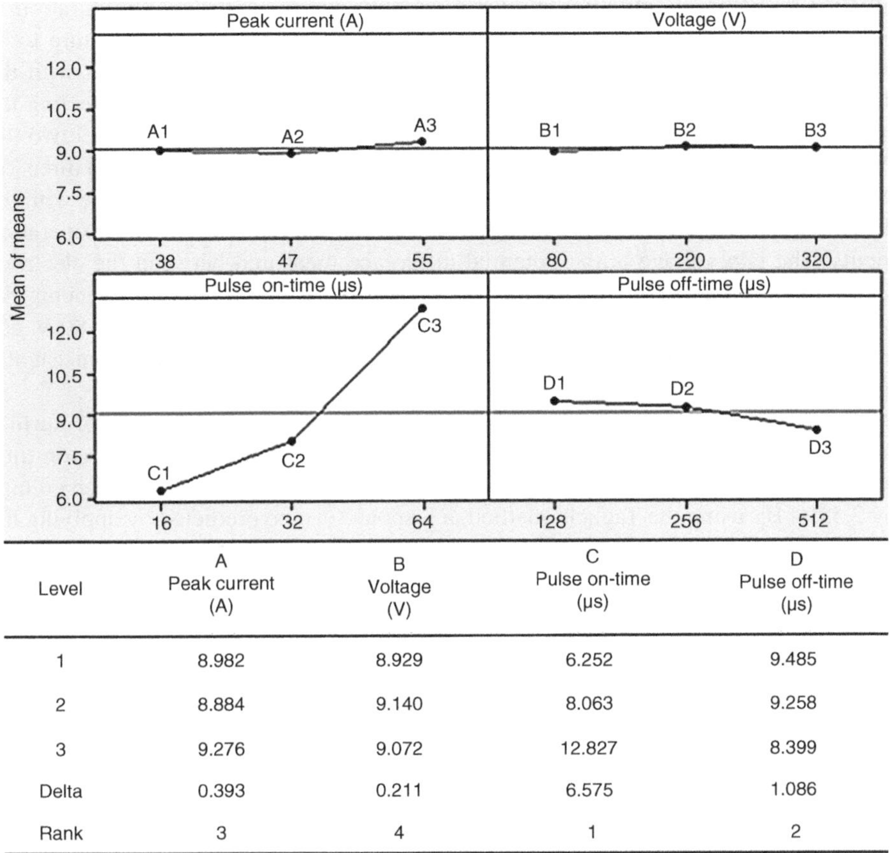

Level	A Peak current (A)	B Voltage (V)	C Pulse on-time (µs)	D Pulse off-time (µs)
1	8.982	8.929	6.252	9.485
2	8.884	9.140	8.063	9.258
3	9.276	9.072	12.827	8.399
Delta	0.393	0.211	6.575	1.086
Rank	3	4	1	2

FIGURE 3.1   C-EDM main effects plot of means with data response of means on surface roughness.

B1, C1, and D3 was predicted to obtain the lowest surface roughness within the limits of the examined level values. On the other hand, the combination of operation inputs value at A3, B2, C3, and D1 was predicted to obtain the highest surface roughness.

Among those four operation inputs, pulse on-time with the delta value of 6.575 µm was identified as the most significant operation input affecting the surface roughness of magnesium alloy machined surface. The results indicate that the pulse on-time was directly proportional to the response. The higher pulse on-time resulting in rougher surface roughness due to longer duration of spark discharging in one cutting cycle and the lower pulse on-time resulting in smoother surface roughness due to the shorter duration of spark discharging in one cutting cycle. The higher pulse on-time permits more materials to be removed in one cutting cycle. It was opposed to the second most significant operation input, pulse off-time with the delta value of 1.086 µm. The results indicate that the lower pulse off-time resulting in rougher surface roughness due to shorter resting duration in one cutting cycle and the higher pulse off-time resulting in smoother surface roughness due to longer resting duration in one cutting cycle. The longer pulse off-time allows the localized temperature to be reduced and better removal of debris from the cutting area. Peak current with the delta value of 0.393 µm was the third most significant operation input affecting the surface roughness of magnesium alloy. In this case, the peak current at level two (47 A) resulting in lower surface roughness and the highest peak current at level three (55 A) resulting in higher surface roughness. On the other hand, the gap voltage with the delta value 0.211 µm was identified less significant compared to the other operation inputs. The gap voltage is the potential difference measured between the electrode and workpiece before any discharge takes place and it is not really influencing the changes of magnesium alloy machined surface roughness. Therefore, the 80 V gap voltage which affects to the lowest surface roughness has been applied consistently in the PM-EDM experiments.

As shown in Figure 3.2, this research encounters that the changes of surface roughness of magnesium alloy machined surface are influenced by the pulse on-time for about 79.55%, pulse off-time by 13.14%, peak current by 4.75%, and gap voltage by 2.55%. By using the Taguchi method, a response can be predicted by applying the Equation (4.3), where $\bar{T}$ is the total mean, $\overline{Ax}$ is the mean of data response of the first operation input, $\overline{Bx}$ is the mean of data response of the second operation input, $\overline{Cx}$ is the mean of data response of the third operation input, and $\overline{Dx}$ is the mean of data response of the fourth operation input.

$$M = \bar{T} + \left(\overline{Ax} - \bar{T}\right) + \left(\overline{Bx} - \bar{T}\right) + \left(\overline{Cx} - \bar{T}\right) + \left(\overline{Dx} - \bar{T}\right) \qquad (3.1)$$

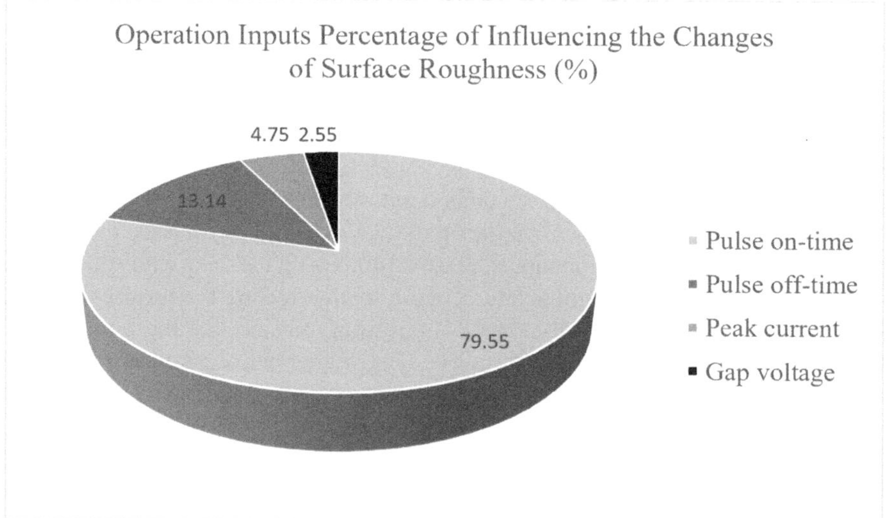

FIGURE 3.2 Operation inputs contribution in affecting the surface roughness of C-EDM experiments.

With the total mean of 9.047 µm, by changing the value of data response of means, the surface roughness of magnesium alloy can be predicted using Equation (4.4), where SR is the surface roughness, $\bar{A}$ is the data response of peak current, $\bar{B}$ is the data response of gap voltage, $\bar{C}$ is the data response of pulse on-time, and $\bar{D}$ is the data response of pulse off-time.

$$SR = 9.047 + \left(\bar{A} - 9.047\right) + \left(\bar{B} - 9.047\right) + \left(\bar{C} - 9.047\right) + \left(\bar{D} - 9.047\right) \qquad (3.2)$$

The optimum combination of C-EDM operation inputs for the smallest surface roughness was selected from the lowest value of each input in the main effects plot of means as presented in Figure 3.1. The inputs are 47 A peak current, 80 V gap voltage, 16 µs pulse on-time, and 512 µs pulse off-time. The predicted surface roughness to be obtained by this combination was computed using Equation (4.4) and the result obtained was 5.322 µm. A confirmation test has been conducted and the actual surface roughness was analyzed. The result obtained was 5.561 µm. It indicates 95.5% similarity to the predicted surface roughness. Therefore, Equation (4.4) was strongly accepted.

If the interaction effects are taken into account, the optimum combination of C-EDM operation inputs for smallest surface roughness are 45.21 A peak current, 88.99 V gap voltage, 16.24 µs pulse on-time, and 506.24 µs pulse off-time. However, the values are not available in the EDM user manual for selection. Therefore, the optimum values obtained from the main effects plot are selected.

The individual effect of each operation input on the surface roughness has been plotted by having the value of the other three operation inputs constant at the lowest level. Figure 3.3 indicates that the highest surface roughness is obtained at 55 A peak current and the lowest surface roughness is obtained at 46 A. However, the nearest value of peak current can be selected in the EDM machine is 47 A.

Figure 3.4 indicates that the highest surface roughness is obtained at 235 V gap voltage and the lowest surface roughness is obtained at 80 V.

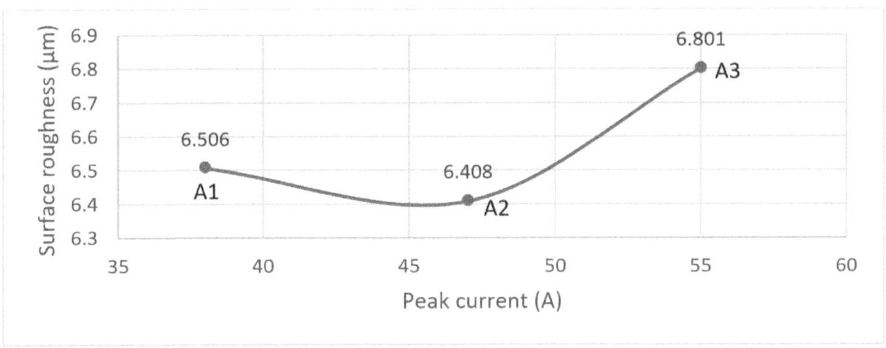

FIGURE 3.3 Individual effect of peak current.

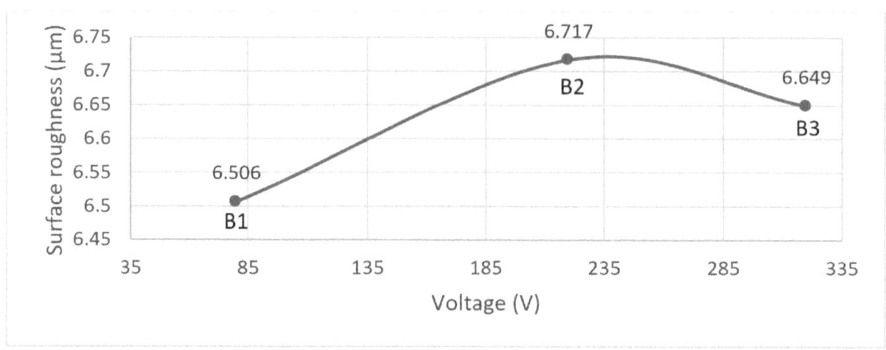

FIGURE 3.4   Individual effect of gap voltage.

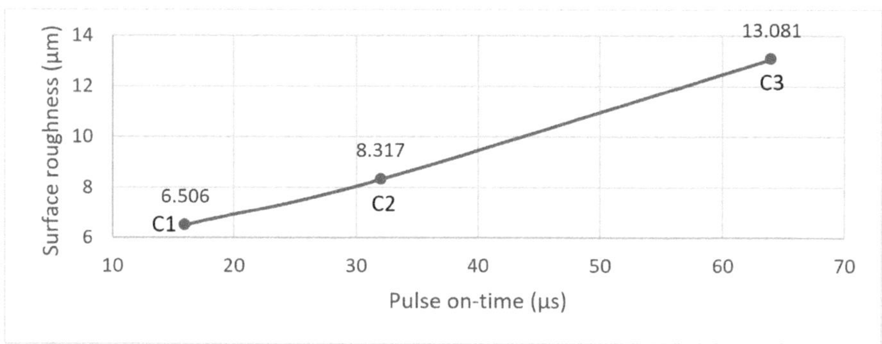

FIGURE 3.5   Individual effect of pulse on-time.

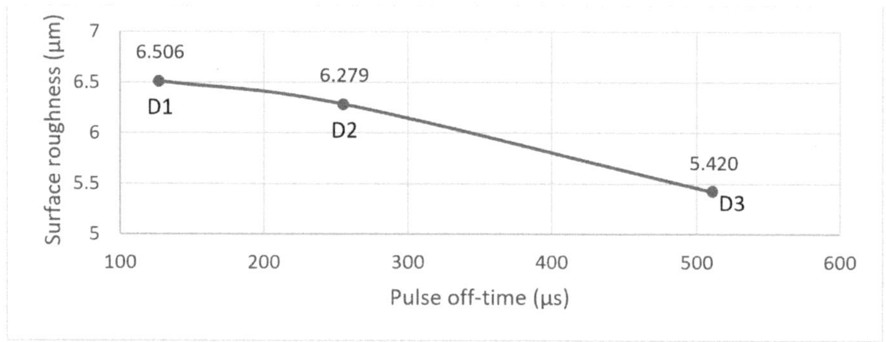

FIGURE 3.6   Individual effect of pulse off-time.

Figure 3.5 indicates that the highest surface roughness is obtained at 64 µs pulse on-time and the lowest surface roughness is obtained at 16 µs. The graph shows that the higher sparking duration resulting in rougher machining surface.

Figure 3.6 indicates that the highest surface roughness is obtained at 128 µs pulse off-time and the lowest surface roughness is obtained at 512 µs. It shows that the higher pulse off-time resulting in smoother machining surface.

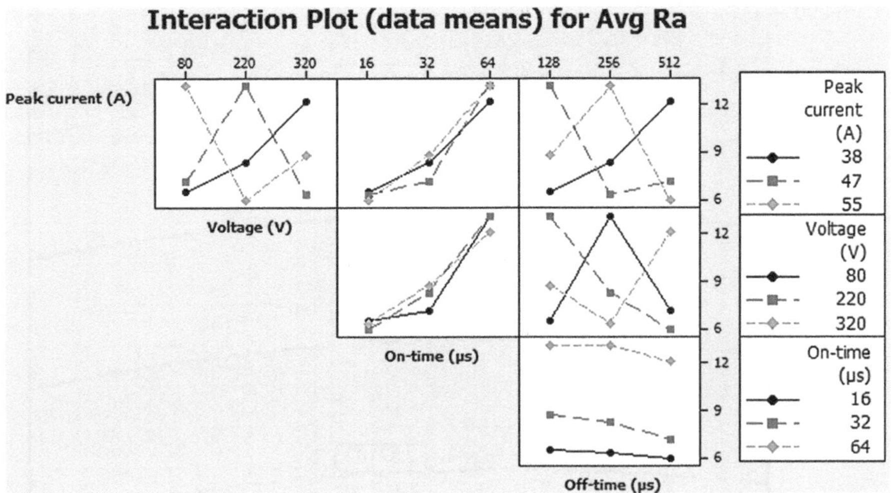

FIGURE 3.7   C-EDM operation inputs interaction plots on the surface roughness.

3.4.1.2   Interaction Plots for Surface Roughness of C-EDM Experiments

Figure 3.7 presents the interaction plots among the operation inputs on the surface roughness. It can be seen that changes in the level of one or two controlled inputs affect the output response. The graph shows that only the effects between pulse on-time and pulse off-time has no interaction. Meanwhile, the pulse on-time which is identified as the most significant operation input set at a lower value resulting in lower surface roughness and vice versa as shown in Figure 3.8. On the other interactions between the operation inputs, the effect of one input depends upon another input. These scenario consequences in no parallel trends in the interaction plot. The spark energy increases with the higher peak current, pulse on-time, and gap voltage which ensuing rougher machined surface.

An operation input is not significantly affecting the response when its p-value is larger than 0.1 in ANOVA. The ANOVA presented in Table 3.4 shows that all interactions between pulse on-time with the other operation inputs is not significant to the response. The significant interactions found are including the peak current with gap voltage which is the most significant interaction, peak current with the pulse off-time and gap voltage with pulse off-time. Even though there are significant interactions found in the ANOVA, it is not necessary to be considered because in the EDM process, selection of any operation input value is limited to the available value provided in the EDM user manual. For instance, the optimized pulse on-time obtained from the operation inputs interaction analysis is 16.24 µs and this value is not available in the EDM user manual. The closest value available for selection is 16 µs.

3.4.1.3   Surface Morphology of C-EDM Experiments

In order to have further understanding of the affected surface structure, SEM images of the machined surfaces were taken and analyzed. Figure 3.9 A presents the SEM

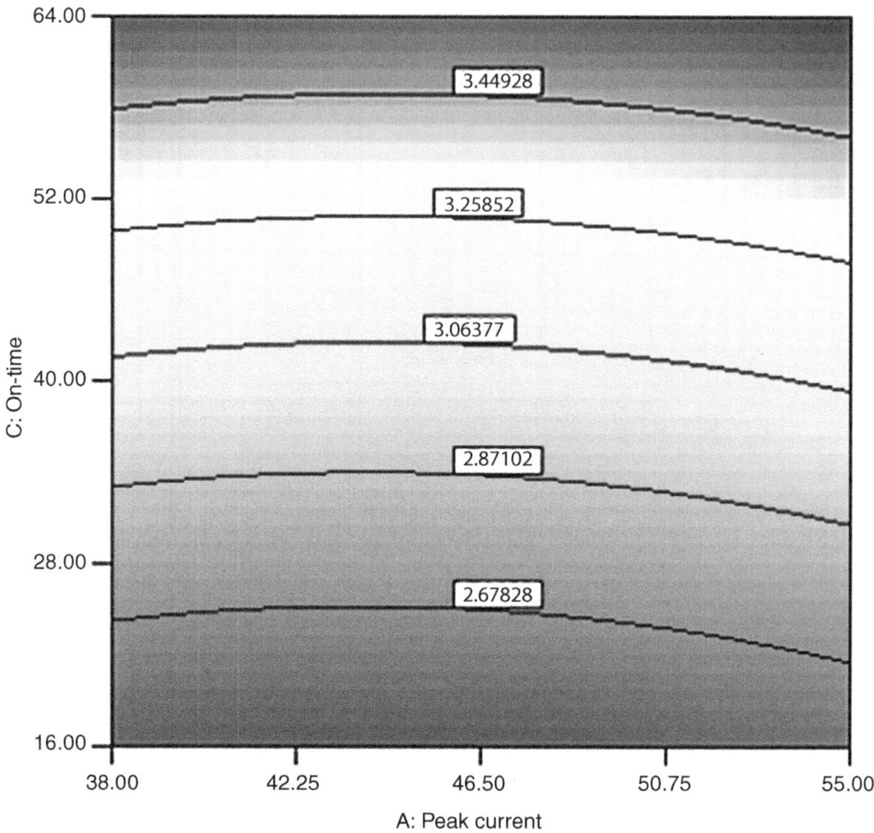

FIGURE 3.8   Interaction between peak current and pulse on-time on the surface roughness.

image of machined surface from experiment 8 (processed with 55 A peak current, 220 V gap voltage, 16 μs pulse on-time, and 512 μs pulse off-time) which obtained the lowest surface roughness. Figure 3.9 B presents the SEM image of machined surface from experiment 5 (processed with 47 A peak current, 220 V gap voltage, 64 μs pulse on-time, and 128 μs pulse off-time) which obtained the highest surface roughness.

As presented in Figure 3.9, the higher surface roughness obtained from the experiment 5 is mainly due to higher peak and deeper ravine. The larger formation of globules and voids can be identified in surface B compared to surface A. Other than that, an obvious micro-crack with the length dimension of 75.3 μm is also found on surface B. The higher pulse on-time and lower pulse off-time applied in experiment 5 results in longer duration of spark discharging and shorter resting duration in one cutting cycle. The longer duration of spark discharging permits more materials to be removed and leave cracks and craters on the machined surface. These formations are not good for biomedical implant application due to direct contact and reaction with body fluid such as water, proteins, and amino acids. In-vitro study reported by Wong et al. shows that the uncoated magnesium alloy corrodes 12 mg per 2 months [15].

TABLE 3.4
ANOVA of C-EDM operation inputs on the surface roughness

Source	Sum of squares	df	Mean square	*F* value	*p*-value
Model	209.92	14	14.99	3.7E+08	<0.0001
A-Peak current	0.3897	1	0.39	9629217	<0.0001
B-Gap voltage	0.0915	1	0.091	2259887	<0.0001
C-Pulse on-time	194.16	1	194.2	4.8E+09	<0.0001
D-Pulse off-time	5.295	1	5.295	1.31E+08	<0.0001
AB	2E-07	1	2E-07	5.762694	0.0373
AC	7E-10	1	7E-10	0.017995	0.8959
AD	2E-07	1	2E-07	5.507084	0.0409
BC	0	1	0	0	1.0000
BD	2E-07	1	2E-07	5.402297	0.0425
CD	0	1	0	0	1.0000
A^2	0.1643	1	0.164	4060328	<0.0001
B^2	0.0413	1	0.041	1020661	<0.0001
C^2	0.363	1	0.363	8967451	<0.0001
D^2	0.0457	1	0.046	1129405	<0.0001
Residual	4E-07	10	4E-08		
Cor total	209.92	24			

Even though magnesium alloy was suggested compatible for temporary implants application, high corrosion rate of the implant causes degradation whilst the defect is yet to be recuperated.

From the EDX spectrum analysis of specimens from the experiments 8 and 5 as presented in Figure 3.10, there are 87.4% magnesium, 4.4% aluminum, and 3.2% zinc discovered from the examined area of experiment 8 specimen and 84.6% magnesium, 6.0% aluminum, and 3.4% zinc are discovered from the examined area of experiment 5 specimen. The difference in weight percentage of the major elements from the experiment 8 as compared to experiment 5 are the experiment 8 specimen machined surface composed of 2.8% more magnesium, 1.6% less aluminum, and 0.2% less zinc.

3.4.2 SURFACE ANALYSIS OF PM-EDM EXPERIMENTS

The roughness of magnesium alloy machined surface may influence its rate of corrosion. Compared to C-EDM method, PM-EDM method is hypothesized to obtain the smoother machined surface. This section discusses the analysis results on the surface roughness of PM-EDM experiments. Table 3.5 presents the average surface roughness values obtained from PM-EDM experiments which were conducted on three specimens for each operation inputs combination and three measurements were taken from each specimen. The lowest surface roughness value was obtained from

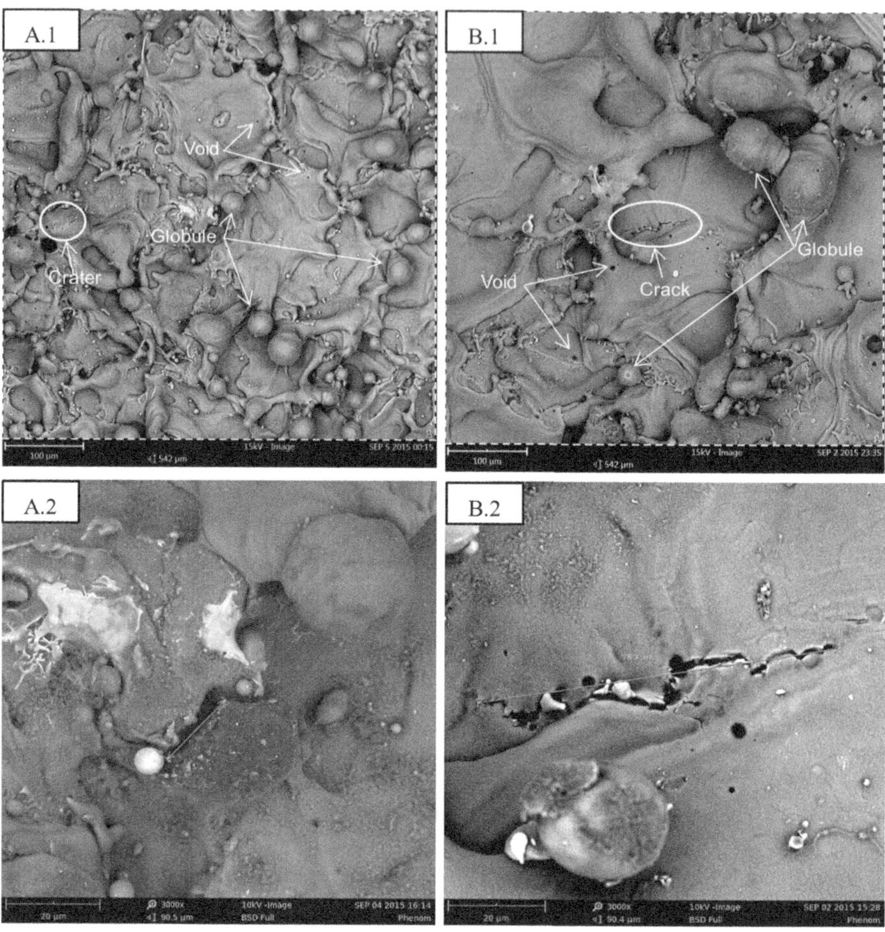

FIGURE 3.9 SEM images; (A) experiment 8 (processed with 55 A peak current, 220 V gap voltage, 16 µs pulse on-time, and 512 µs pulse off-time) and (B) experiment 5 (processed with 47 A peak current, 220 V gap voltage, 64 µs pulse on-time, and 128 µs pulse off-time).

the experiment 6 with 4.873 µm. The operation inputs combination of experiment 6 were 2 g/l powder concentration, 55 A peak current, 16 µs pulse on-time, and 256 µs pulse off-time. On the other hand, the highest surface roughness value was obtained from experiment 5 with 13.428 µm. The operation inputs combination of experiment 5 were 2 g/l powder concentration, 47 A peak current, 64 µs pulse on-time, and 128 µs pulse off-time. Based on the collected data, earlier assumption that can be made was that the concentration of conductive particles has a less significant effect on the surface roughness compared to the other operation inputs. This was because both the lowest and highest surface roughness were obtained from the experiments with 2 g/ l powder concentration.

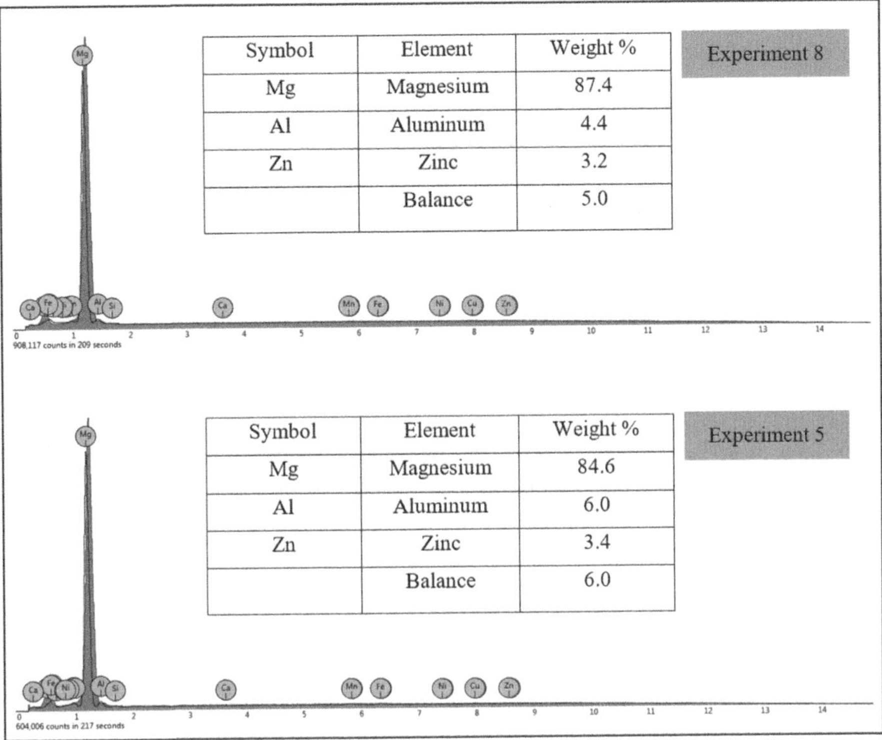

FIGURE 3.10 EDX spectrum of machined surface from experiment 8 (processed with 55 A peak current, 220 V gap voltage, 16 µs pulse on-time, and 512 µs pulse off-time) and experiment 5 (processed with 47 A peak current, 220 V gap voltage, 64 µs pulse on-time, and 128 µs pulse off-time).

TABLE 3.5
Surface roughness of PM-EDM experiments

| | Controlled operation inputs | | | | Surface roughness (µm) | | | |
Exp.	Powder concentration (g/l)	Peak current (A)	Pulse on-time (µs)	Pulse off-time (µs)	Specimen 1	Specimen 2	Specimen 3	Average
1	1	38	16	128	5.474	5.667	6.192	5.778
2	1	47	32	256	8.106	7.102	8.106	7.771
3	1	55	64	512	12.641	13.733	13.587	13.320
4	2	38	32	512	6.421	6.304	7.002	6.576
5	2	47	64	128	17.113	12.649	10.521	13.428
6	2	55	16	256	5.019	4.885	4.715	4.873
7	3	38	64	256	10.605	10.620	10.400	10.542
8	3	47	16	512	5.555	5.634	5.279	5.489
9	3	55	32	128	9.833	11.662	9.651	10.382

3.4.2.1 Main Effects Plot on the Surface Roughness of PM-EDM Experiments

The collected data from PM-EDM experiments were further analyzed using the Taguchi method. The main effects plot with data response of means indicates that the most significant operation input affecting the surface roughness is pulse on-time with the delta value of 7.050 µm and followed by pulse off-time with the delta value of 2.134 µm. The peak current ranked at third with the delta value of 1.893 µm. These ranks are similar to the one obtained in C-EDM experiments. The zinc powder concentration is ranked at fourth with the delta value of 0.664 µm. Even though the other three operation inputs in PM-EDM experiments were indicated more significant affecting the surface roughness as presented in Figure 3.11, the addition of zinc particles in the PM-EDM experiment did consequence into positive effect on the surface quality. The result presented in Figure 3.11 shows that among three different zinc

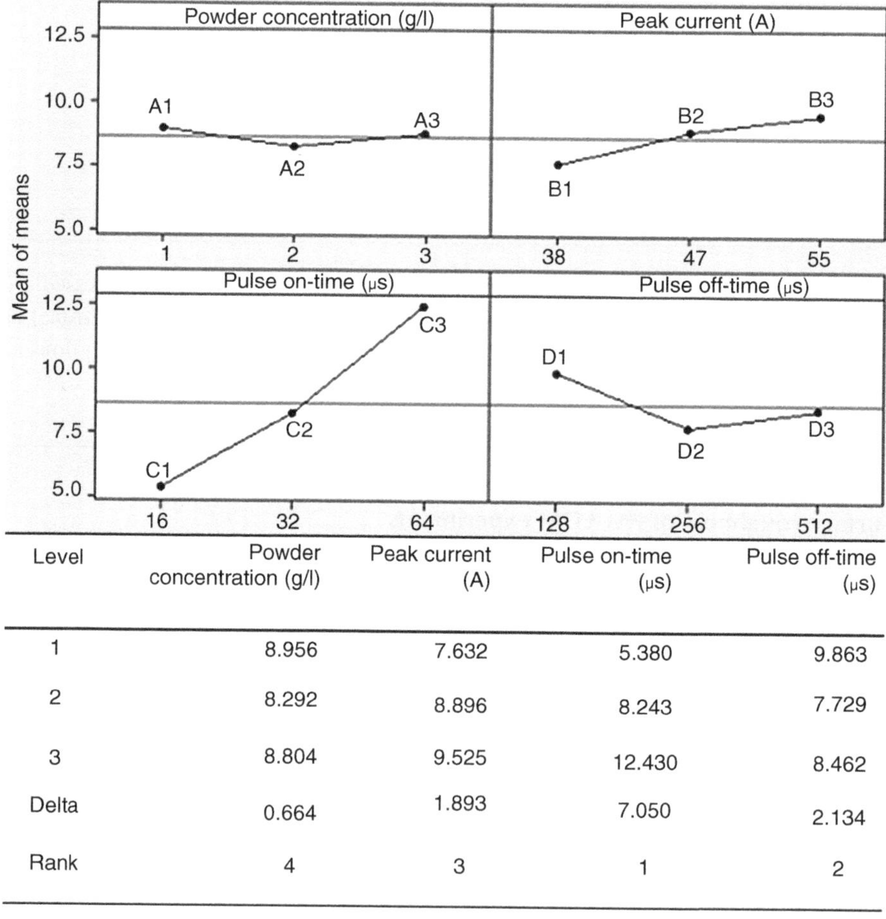

Level	Powder concentration (g/l)	Peak current (A)	Pulse on-time (µs)	Pulse off-time (µs)
1	8.956	7.632	5.380	9.863
2	8.292	8.896	8.243	7.729
3	8.804	9.525	12.430	8.462
Delta	0.664	1.893	7.050	2.134
Rank	4	3	1	2

FIGURE 3.11 PM-EDM main effects plot with data response of means on surface roughness.

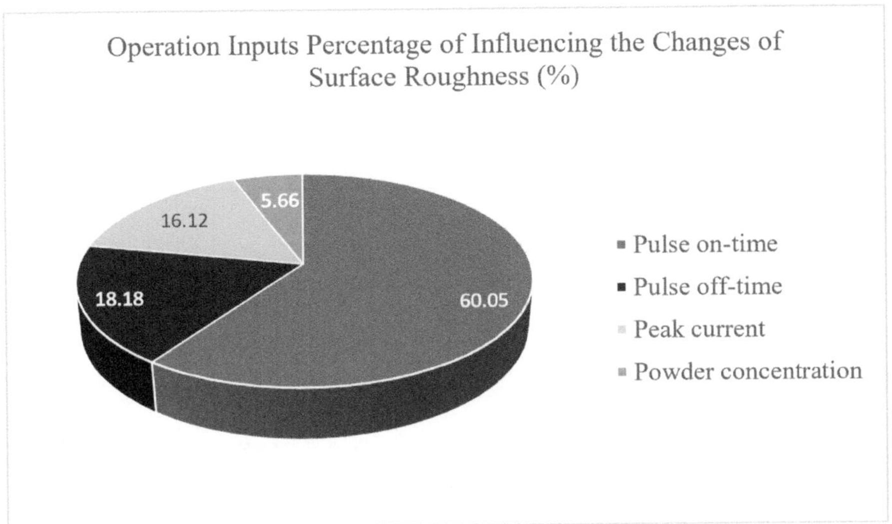

FIGURE 3.12 Operation inputs contribution in affecting the surface roughness of PM-EDM experiments.

TABLE 3.6
Surface roughness of magnesium alloy machined surface processed by C-EDM and PM-EDM method

Exp.	Powder concentration (g/l)	Peak current (A)	Voltage (V)	On-time (µs)	Off-time (µs)	Surface roughness (µm)			
						1	2	3	Average
C-EDM	-	38	80	16	128	6.889	6.393	6.237	6.506
PM-EDM	1	38	80	16	128	5.474	5.667	6.192	5.778

powder concentration, the 2 g/l powder concentration results in the lowest surface roughness. It was aligned with the result obtained by Jabbaripour et al. [16]. The suspended zinc particles in the dielectric fluid specifically in the gap between the electrode and workpiece were influencing the uniformity of the electric sparks' distribution. It improves the ignition distortion and stabilizes the sparks.

As presented in Figure 3.12, the results analysis of PM-EDM experiments encounter that the changes of surface roughness of magnesium alloy machined surface are influenced by the pulse on-time for about 60.05%, pulse off-time by 18.18%, peak current by 16.12%, and powder concentration by 5.66%. Compared to C-EDM method, the PM-EDM method obtained better surface roughness. Results on the surface roughness from experiment 1 of both the C-EDM and PM-EDM are presented in Table 3.6. The same operation inputs of 38 A peak current, 80 V gap voltage, 16 µs pulse on-time, and 128 µs pulse off-time were applied in both experiments. The conducted experiments proved that PM-EDM method has reduced the magnesium

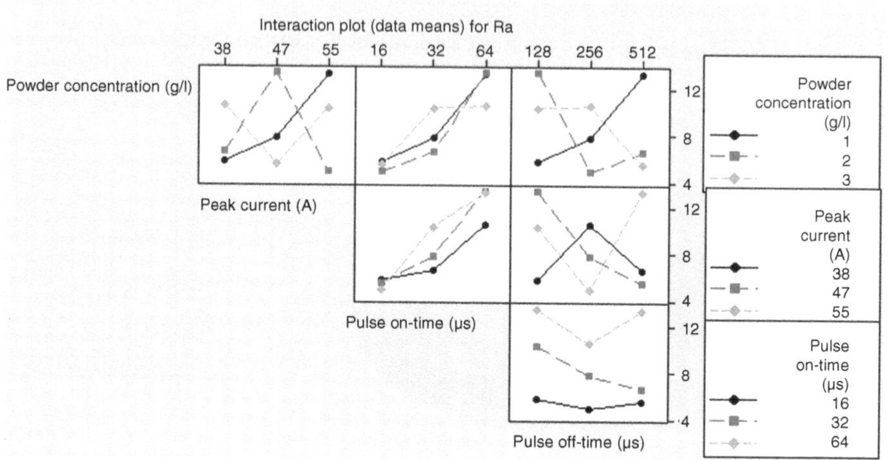

FIGURE 3.13   PM-EDM operation inputs interaction plots on surface roughness.

alloy machined surface roughness by 11.2% compared to C-EDM method. The PM-EDM method is better for fabricating biomedical implants where the quality of machining surface is extremely important.

3.4.2.2   Interaction Plot on the Surface Roughness of PM-EDM Experiments

Figure 3.13 presents the interaction effects of the operation inputs and it can be seen that the changes in the level of any operation input affect the output response. There were interactions that occurred between any two operation inputs except between the pulse on-time and pulse off-time. The effect of one operation input depends upon another operation input. The spark energy increases with increase of peak current and pulse on-time made the machined surface rougher. The metal removal was directly proportionate to the amount of energy applied during the pulse on-time. This energy was controlled by the peak current and duration of pulse on-time. The longer the pulse on-time sustained, the more materials to be melted and removed. The larger pulse on-time produces broader and deeper craters than the craters produced by the shorter pulse on-time. These larger craters resulting in a rougher surface finish.

REFERENCES

[1] M. Razak, A. Rani, N. Saad, G. Littlefair, and A. Aliyu, "Controlling corrosion rate of Magnesium alloy using powder mixed electrical discharge machining," in IOP Conference Series: Materials Science and Engineering, 2018, pp. 1–10.

[2] M. A. H. A. Razak and A. M. Abdul-Rani, "Innovative surface engineering technique for surface modification of Mg alloy for orthopedic application," in Biomanufacturing, ed: Springer, 2019, pp. 225–240.

[3] M. A. Razak, A. M. Abdul-Rani, T. V. V. L. N. Rao, S. R. Pedapati, and S. Kamal, "Electrical discharge machining on biodegradable AZ31 magnesium alloy using Taguchi method," *Procedia Engineering,* vol. 148, pp. 916–922, 2016.

[4] D. K. Singh, *Fundamentals of Manufacturing Engineering*: CRC Press, 2008.

[5] H.-D. Nguyen-Tran, H.-S. Oh, S.-T. Hong, H. N. Han, J. Cao, S.-H. Ahn, *et al.*, "A review of electrically-assisted manufacturing," *International Journal of Precision Engineering and Manufacturing-Green Technology,* vol. 2, pp. 365–376, 2015.

[6] M. A. Razak, A. M. Abdul-Rani, and A. M. Nanimina, "Improving EDM efficiency with silicon carbide powder-mixed dielectric fluid," *International Journal of Materials, Mechanics and Manufacturing,* vol. 3, pp. 40–43, 2015.

[7] V. T. Le, T. L. Banh, X. T. Tran, and N. Thi Hong Minh, "Surface modification process by electrical discharge machining with tungsten carbide powder mixing in kerosene fluid," in *Applied Mechanics and Materials*, 2019, pp. 115–122.

[8] F. Modica, V. Marrocco, and I. Fassi, "Micro-electro-discharge machining (Micro-EDM)," in *Micro-Manufacturing Technologies and Their Applications*, ed: Springer, 2017, pp. 149–173.

[9] D. K. Naik, A. Khan, H. Majumder, and R. K. Garg, "Experimental investigation of the PMEDM of nickel free austenitic stainless steel: a promising coronary stent material," *Silicon,* vol. 11, pp. 899–907, 2019.

[10] D. Hanaoka, Y. Fukuzawa, C. Ramirez, P. Miranzo, M. Osendi, and M. Belmonte, "Electrical discharge machining of ceramic/carbon nanostructure composites," *Procedia CIRP,* vol. 6, pp. 95–100, 2013.

[11] S.-F. Ou and C.-Y. Wang, "Effects of bioceramic particles in dielectric of powder-mixed electrical discharge machining on machining and surface characteristics of titanium alloys," *Journal of Materials Processing Technology,* vol. 245, pp. 70–79, 2017.

[12] R. Bajaj, A. K. Tiwari, and A. R. Dixit, "Current trends in electric discharge machining using micro and nano powder materials-a review," *Materials Today: Proceedings,* vol. 2, pp. 3302–3307, 2015.

[13] N. Kumar, P. Ale, N. Kumar, and S. Sharma, "Study of PMEDM efficiency on HCHCr steel using silicon powder in dielectric fluid," *International Journal of Emerging Technologies in Engineering Research,* vol. 4, pp. 54–61, 2016.

[14] A. Abdul-Rani, M. Razak, G. Littlefair, I. Gibson, and A. Nanimina, "Improving EDM process on AZ31 magnesium alloy towards sustainable biodegradable implant manufacturing," *Procedia Manufacturing,* vol. 7, pp. 504–509, 2016.

[15] H. M. Wong, K. W. Yeung, K. O. Lam, V. Tam, P. K. Chu, K. D. Luk, *et al.*, "A biodegradable polymer-based coating to control the performance of magnesium alloy orthopaedic implants," *Biomaterials,* vol. 31, pp. 2084–2096, 2010.

[16] B. Jabbaripour, M. H. Sadeghi, M. R. Shabgard, and H. Faraji, "Investigating surface roughness, material removal rate and corrosion resistance in PMEDM of γ-TiAl intermetallic," *Journal of Manufacturing Processes,* vol. 15, pp. 56–68, 2013.

4 Innovative Biomimetic Electro-Discharge Coating on Bulk Metallic Glass for Potential Orthopedic Application

Abdul Azeez Abdu Aliyu, Ahmad Majdi Abdul-Rani, Iqtidar Ahmed Gul, Elhuseini Garba, Tang Tong Boon, Nabihah Bt Sallih, and Sadaqat Ali

4.1 INTRODUCTION

Metallic glasses (MGs) are non-crystalline or amorphous class of advanced materials. The first MGs (Au75Si25), also called liquid metals or amorphous alloys, were first discovered in 1960 by Duwez at Caltech, USA through rapid quenching technique [1]. MGs have outstanding physical, chemical, and mechanical behaviors such as high resistance to corrosion and high toughness, when compared with Ti alloys [2–7]. Rapid rise in researches on MGs was noticed between 1970s and 1980s following the discovery of continuous casting for fabrication of commercial MGs ribbons, lines, and sheets [8]. The discovery of higher glass formers elements such as Pd, Ni, Be, Al, etc., led to the development and production of MGs into larger size (up to 10 mm diameter and 100 mm long) called bulk metallic glasses (BMGs) [9]. The emergence of BMGs overcomes the limitations of MGs. A series of BMGs of either Zr-, Mg-, La-, Pd-, Ti-, and Fe-based were discovered in the early 1990s through conventional mold casting by Caltech group [10, 11]. The first commercial BMG material called Vitreloy 1 in the form of Zr41.2Ti13.8Cu12.5Ni10Be22.5 was discovered in 1992 by Johnson and Peker. Further studies by Axinte [12] investigated some Zr-based BMG with high glass-forming like Vit105 represented by Zr52.5Ti5Cu17.9Ni14.6Al10.

Various conventional and non-conventional shaping techniques have been employed to produce BMG components for several applications [13]. Thermoplastic process, blow molding, capacitive discharge forming, selective laser die casting, and end casting were some classic techniques used in shaping BMG to produce some components. It exists, some few recent researches on the EDM of BMG, to determine the capability of EDM process to cut BMG without much influence on its initial performance [14–17]. Severe crystallization of BMG on its surface was noticed,

DOI: 10.1201/9781003456018-4

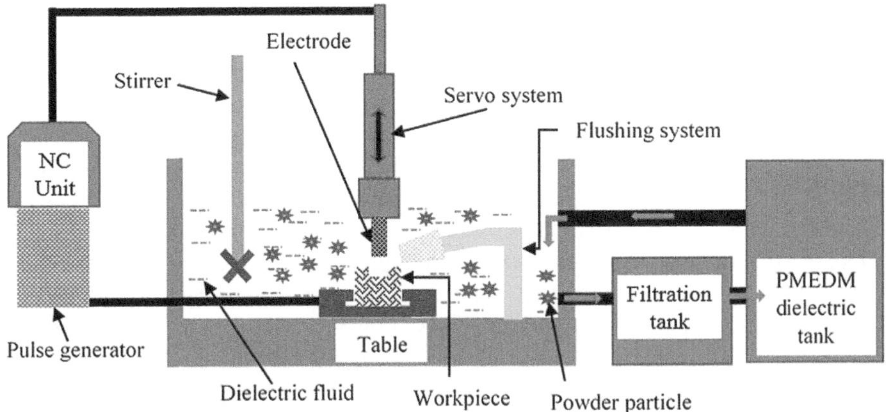

FIGURE 4.1   Schematic diagram of complete AM-EDM experimental-set up.

especially when high energy is used [18, 19]. Addition of substances to the dielectric fluid, refer to as additive-mixed EDM (AM-EDM) is considered the most promising approach for modifying the surface of the workpiece [17]. Figure 4.1 shows a complete schematic diagram of AM-EDM.

AM-EDM is a novel technique which can be used to deposit a bioceramic biocompatible, and bioactive oxide layer on the implant surface. Recently, the potential application of AM-EDM for the surface treatment of Ti-based metallic implant has been reported by Prakash et al. [20]. The nano-porous bioceramic layer was deposited on the Ti-substrate to enhance its micro-hardness, corrosion resistance, and in-vitro bioactivity [21]. The bone–implant interface strength was found very sound when the implant surface was treated by AM-EDM process [22]. A nanoporous and calcium-rich oxide layer is produced on Ti-6Al-4V surface when 0.1 Mol/l of calcium chloride aqueous solution was added into deionized water during sinking EDM [23]. This oxide surface was proved to have high hardness and reasonable biocompatibility, enough for biomedical applications, especially for bone and teeth implant.

In this study, different concentration of HA powder was added into the dielectric fluid during the AM-EDM of Zr-based BMG, with aim to enhance the surface strength, biocompatibility, and osteointegration of the Zr-based BMG surface as a potential implant. Various microstructures and phases that formed on the coated Zr-based BMG was investigated. The formation of a biomimetic oxide and carbide coating synthesized on the Zr-based BMG surface by hydroxyapatite AM-EDM process was ascertained.

4.2   MATERIALS AND METHODS

4.2.1   Sample Preparation

The optical microscope (Model: LEICA, NICON) and SEM facilities was used to investigate the coated layer on the Zr-based BMG. The sample preparation involved various stages. In the first stage, the cross-section of the coated Zr-based BMG specimen is mounted using automatic mounting press (Model: Simpliment 1000). The samples are normally mounted to enable ease of handling during grinding/polishing operations. In the second stage, the mounted sample was ground metaserv 250 grinder-polisher using SiC grits grinding papers. The grinding operation was carried out in five stages using 180, 400, 600, 800, and 1200 grades of SiC abrasive grinding papers. The polishing was also made by metaserv 250 grinder–polisher instrument in four stages using 3, 2, 1, and 0.05 μm-sized polycrystalline diamond suspension. The last stage of sample preparation is the etching process. The etchant solution of 2 ml HNO_3, 2 ml HF, and 96 ml distilled water was prepared as done by Rafique [24]. The mirror-like polished specimens were immersed into the prepared etchant solution for 15 s. At this time, the samples were removed from the etchant and apply some drops of ethanol to stop the etching process. The etched specimens were then observed in the optical microscope to confirm the presence of the coating in the specimens. Upon a successful coating on the etched Zr-based BMG specimens, a further analysis using SEM instrument was carried out.

4.2.2 SURFACE MORPHOLOGY

During EDM/HA-EDM process, the treated surface undergoes various changes due to spark and material deposition on the substrate material surface. However, the surface of the Zr-based BMG material is melted and quenched immediately by the flowing dielectric fluid. This resulted in various metallurgical and chemical changes on the treated Zr-based BMG surface. Thus, proper investigation of the surface morphology of the treated material is a key concern in this research. Surface morphology investigation enables us to observe some defects such as micro-cracks, voids, craters, etc., on the treated Zr-based BMG. However, the nature, distribution, and size of the porosities that might be produced during EDM/HA-EDM process can be investigated. SEM (Model: SEM, Evo LS15) was used to investigate the surface morphology and pores formation of the machined and coated Zr-based BMG surface. During EDM/HA-EDM process, suspended powder and tool-electrode materials are expected to be transferred and deposited on the treated Zr-based BMG surface. This material might be deposited in elemental or compound form. Therefore, the chemical elements deposited on the Zr-based BMG specimen investigation is of great interest in this research. SEM and X-ray photoelectron spectroscopy (XPS) facilities were employed to investigate and analyze the elements' presence on the treated and untreated specimens.

4.2.3 PHASE/COMPOUNDS (XRD) ANALYSIS

The primary function of XRD is to identify crystalline phases of a compound and determine the unit cell dimension. XRD is a non-destructive test which is also used to determine the crystal structure, crystal orientation, the average grain size, crystallinity, strain, and crystal defects. The mechanism of its operation involves setting of a monochromatic beam of X-rays diffracted at specific angles from lattice planes (specimen), thereby producing the XRD peaks. The distribution of atoms in a lattice provides the peak intensity. The XRD pattern of a given specimen is a fingerprint of its periodic arrangement. EDM/HA-EDM process which involved heating, melting, vaporization, and subsequent solidification of workpiece and tool materials, resulted in material deposition on the substrate material. This leads to several phase changes and transformation on the treated Zr-based BMG surface. The XRD pattern of the treated Zr-based BMG specimens was examined at scanning range of $2\theta = 20°\text{–}90°$ and step size of 0.01°/step size.

4.3　RESULTS AND DISCUSSIONS

4.3.1　Surface Morphology Analysis

The FESEM micrograph shown in Figure 4.2 depicts the formation of the HA coatings on the treated BMG matrix. Two distinct phases could be noticed, a dark HA coating containing oxide/carbide phases, which covers almost half of the machined surface and a light BMG phase as presented in Figure 4.2a. Various nanocracks, nanopores, and some debris could be observed. The phenomenon of oxide/carbide phase formation on the Zr-based BMG surface during HA-EDM process could be explained by the mechanism of material migration. During the spark, materials from the CpTi

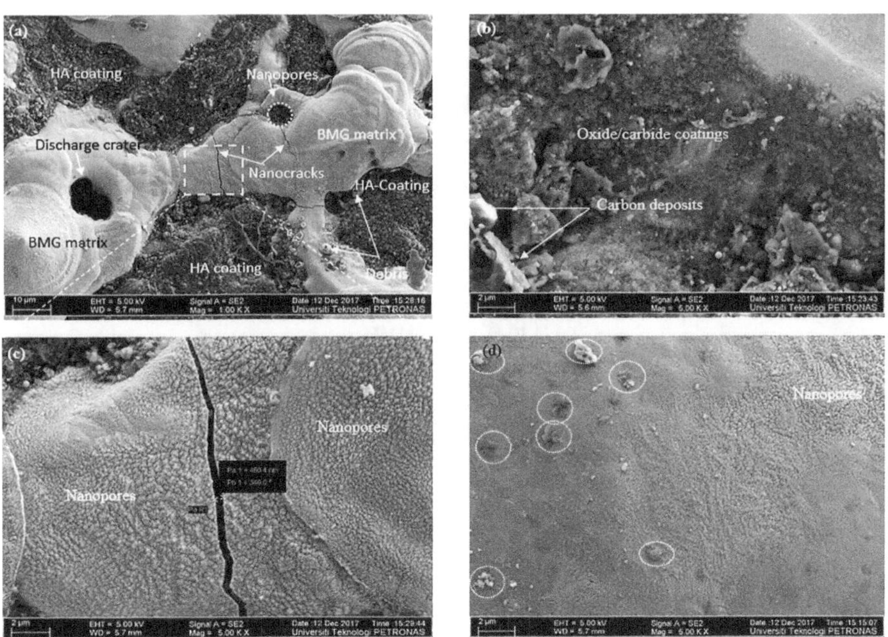

FIGURE 4.2　Oxide and carbide coating formation on the HA-EDMed (8 A, 4 µs, 15 g/l). (a) HA and BMG phases, (b) oxide/carbide phases, (c) BMG phase and (d) nano-crack on the BMG matrix.

tool-electrode and the suspended HA powder are melted, vaporized, and migrated to the Zr-based BMG surface in elemental or compound form. During the off-time, that is, a resting period before next cycle, the Ca and O from the decomposed HA powder $(Ca_5(PO4)_3OH)$ fuse to the Zr from Zr-Cu-Ni-Ti-Be BMG substrate material and solidifies on the BMG matrix, forming a calcium-enriched, nanoporous bioceramic oxides, and hard carbide coatings. At 5000× magnification, a rough oxide and carbide films, and some carbon deposit could be observed in Figure 4.2b. A nano-size crack measured about 400 nm was also noticed as shown in Figure 4.2c. The crack might occur due to the high discharge current and the rapid quenching of the melted Zr-based BMG surface. Some debris, which occurred due to re-solidification of the unwashed melted BMG were present in the BMG matrix (encircled in red) as presented in Figure 4.2d.

4.3.2 COATING LAYERS

To determine the HA coating thickness deposited by HA-EDM process on the Zr-based BMG surface, the cross-section of the treated specimens was observed through SEM. The HA-coated Zr-based BMG shows three distinct layers as elaborated in Figure 4.3. The top recast layer which is formed due to unflushed re-solidified debris. This layer has low adhesion strength and can easily be polished. Next layer is the hard nanostructured and nanoporous bioceramic oxide and carbide coatings. This layer

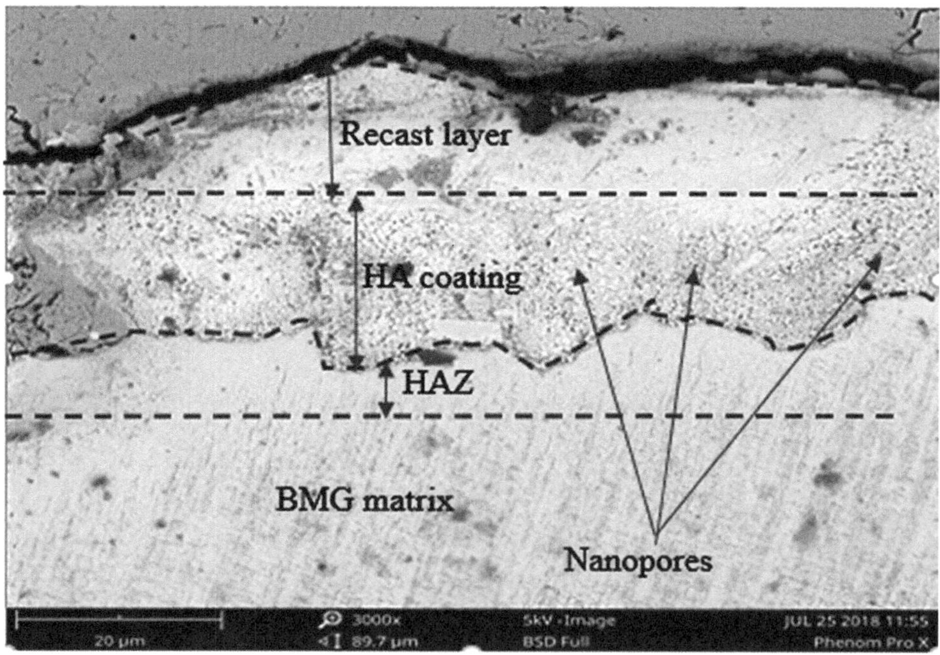

FIGURE 4.3   Cross-section of the HA-coated Zr-based BMG by HA-EDM process.

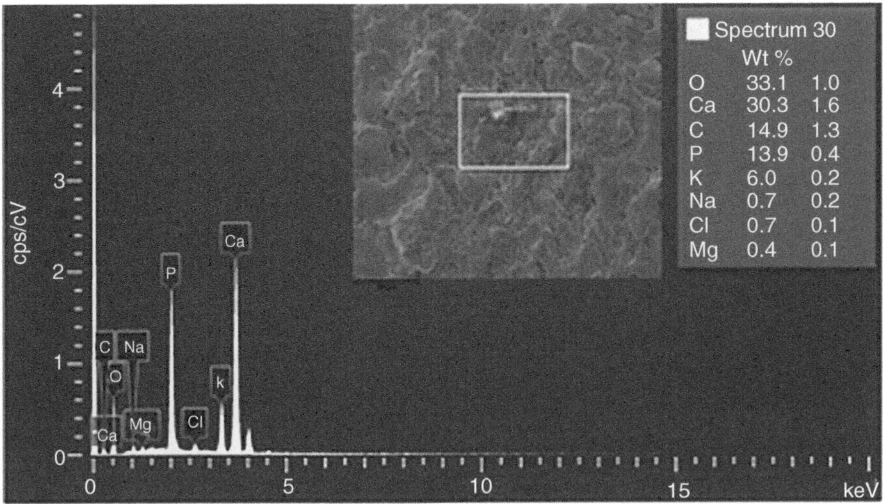

FIGURE 4.4 EDX spectrum of the HA-coated Zr-based BMG specimen by HA-EDM process.

is produced from the HA and Zr-Ti-Cu-Ni-Be BMG elemental constituents, which melt, react, and solidify on the Zr-based BMG matrix. Last layer is the heat affected zone, a layer which is heated but not melted. It was also observed that the coating formed is not uniform.

4.3.3 Elemental Deposition Analysis

The energy-dispersive X-ray (EDX) spectrum shown in Figure 4.4 depicted the presence of various HA elements on the coated Zr-based BMG by HA-EDM process. The elemental distribution observed in spectrum 30 shows the deposition of 33.1 wt% O, 30.3 wt% Ca, 14.9 wt% C, 13.9 wt% P, 6.0 wt% K, 0.7 wt% Na, 0.7 wt% Cl, and 0.4 wt% Mg on the coated Zr-based BMG surface. This confirmed the capability of HA-EDM process to deposit HA on the Zr-based BMG surface. Some foreign elements such as Na, Cl, and Mg might initially be present as trace elements in the HA. Furthermore, these elements are non-toxic to the body [25].

4.3.4 Bioceramic Oxides and Carbides Phases

The XRD patterns of the HA-EDMed Zr-based BMG are presented in Figure 4.5. The samples were treated at a different HA powder concentration (5, 15, and 20 g/L). A predominant broad bump of amorphous Zr-based BMG phase and some crystalline sharp peaks of HA, ZrO_2, $CaZrO_3$, ZrC, and TiC could be observed. The presence of unknown compounds phase was also noticed. The HA phase, which occurs at $2\theta = 35°$, 58°, and 83° is probably due to undecomposed HA powder in the dielectric fluids. However, some of the HA powder in the coating zone is melted and decomposed to

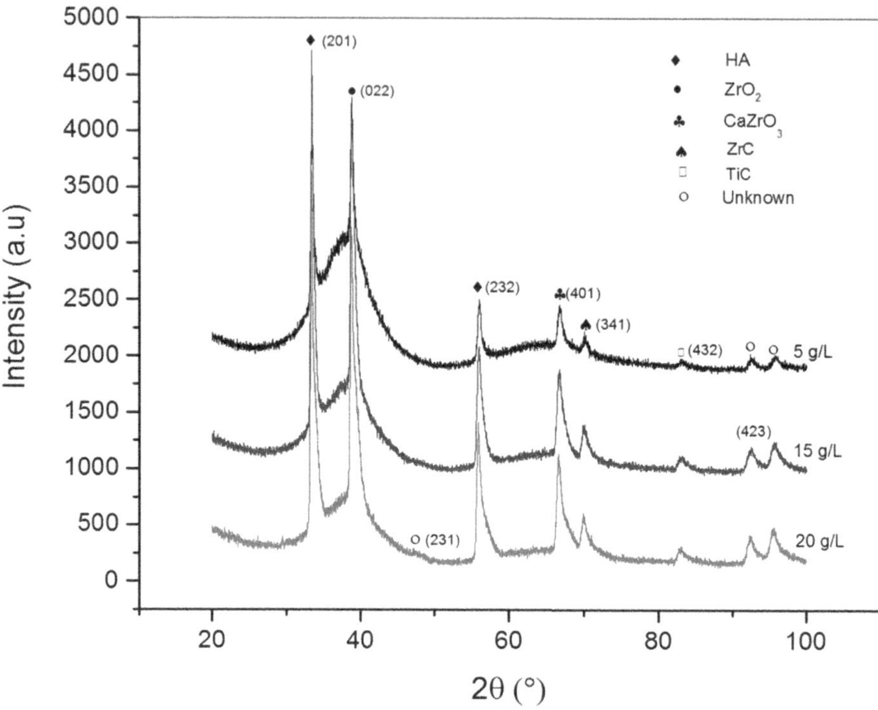

FIGURE 4.5 XRD pattern of the HA-EDM BMG at different powder concentrations (5, 10, and 15 g/L) and constant discharge current of 5 A.

various elements such as Ca, P, O, and K. Ca and O obtained from the decomposed HA reacted with Zr in the Zr-Ti-Cu-Ni-Be BMG and produced a bioceramic oxide like $CaZrO_3$ and ZrO_2. Oxides such $CaZrO_3$, HA, and ZrO_2 are appetite inducers which is believed to enhance the biocompatibility and osteointegration of an implant [26]. Carbide phases such as ZrC and TiC are formed due to reaction of Zr and Ti (tool-electrode) with carbon in the hydrocarbon dielectric fluid. The peaks in XRD pattern of the specimen processed at 20 g/L HA powder concentration are longer and sharper compared to those treated at 15 and 5 g/L. This may be due to high HA powder deposition, which is crystalline in nature.

4.4 CONCLUSION

The experimental result revealed that the coating of about 27.2 μm thick was successfully deposited on the Zr-based BMG material by HA-EDC process. The voltage of about 20 V at a frequency of 5 kHz applied between the tool and the workpiece electrodes provides a sufficient current to ignite the spark at the cutting zone. The Ca and O supplied by the added HA (Ca5(PO4)3OH) powder reacted with the Zr in the Zr-Cu-Ni-Ti-Be BMG workpiece material, thereby producing a biocompatible and bioactive calcium-based bioceramic oxide coating in the form of CaZrO3, CaTiO3,

CaO2 on the Zr-based BMG surface. Furthermore, the burning and decomposition of hydrocarbon-based dielectric fluid liberated C which combines with the Zr and Ti in the electrodes to form an extremely hard ZrC and TiC coatings on the HA-EDCed BMG surface. In addition, the FESEM microstructural study confirmed the formation of numerous dendritic nanostructured surfaces and densely nanoporosities, which are responsible for the enhanced osteointegration of the treated Zr-based BMG material. Moreover, the EDX and XPS analysis confirmed the migration of various HA elements to the Zr-based BMG surface. Elements such as Ca, O, P, and K with a proportion of 30.3, 33.1, 13.9, and 6.0 weight%, respectively, were found present on the coated Zr-based BMG surface. Furthermore, the initial Ni and Be content in the BMG material were completely replaced by these HA elements. This contributed immensely in improving the biocompatibility of the coated Zr-based BMG material.

ACKNOWLEDGMENTS

The authors appreciated the financial support by UP-UTP international collaborative research fund with cost centers 015ME0-081 and 015LB0-040 for supporting this research.

REFERENCES

[1] Jun, W.K., R. Willens, and P. Duwez, Non-crystalline structure in solidified gold–silicon alloys. *Nature*, 1960. 187(4740): p. 869.

[2] Sun, Y., et al., In vitro and in vivo biocompatibility of an Ag-bearing Zr-based bulk metallic glass for potential medical use. *Journal of Non-Crystalline Solids*, 2015. 419: p. 82–91.

[3] Aliyu, A.A.A., et al., Electro-discharge machining of Zr67Cu11Ni10Ti9Be3: An investigation on hydroxyapatite deposition and surface roughness. *Processes*, 2020. 8(6): p. 635.

[4] Schroers, J., et al., Precious bulk metallic glasses for jewelry applications. *Materials Science and Engineering: A*, 2007. 449: p. 235–238.

[5] Schroers, J., et al., Gold based bulk metallic glass. *Applied Physics Letters*, 2005. 87(6): p. 061912.

[6] Tantavisut, S., et al., The novel toxic free titanium-based amorphous alloy for bio-medical application. *Journal of Materials Research and Technology*, 2018. 7(3): p. 248–253.

[7] Tantavisut, S., et al., In vitro biocompatibility of novel titanium-based amorphous alloy thin film in human osteoblast like cells. *Chulalongkorn Medical Journal*, 2019. 63(2): p. 89–93.

[8] Wang, W.-H., C. Dong, and C. Shek, Bulk metallic glasses. *Materials Science and Engineering: R: Reports*, 2004. 44(2): p. 45–89.

[9] Hofmann, D.C., Bulk metallic glasses and their composites: a brief history of diverging fields. *Journal of Materials*, 2013. 2013.

[10] Johnson, W.L., Bulk glass-forming metallic alloys: Science and technology. *MRS Bulletin*, 1999. 24(10): p. 42–56.

[11] Inoue, A. and N. Nishiyama, New bulk metallic glasses for applications as magnetic-sensing, chemical, and structural materials. *MRS Bulletin*, 2007. 32(8): p. 651–658.

[12] Axinte, E., Metallic glasses from "alchemy" to pure science: present and future of design, processing and applications of glassy metals. *Materials & Design*, 2012. 35: p. 518–556.

[13] Axinte, E., et al. An overview on the conventional and nonconventional methods for manufacturing the metallic glasses. In *MATEC Web of Conferences*. 2017. EDP Sciences, France.

[14] Al-Amin, M., et al., Powder mixed-EDM for potential biomedical applications: a critical review. *Materials and Manufacturing Processes*, 2020. 35(16): p. 1789–1811.

[15] Al-Amin, M., et al., Bio-ceramic coatings adhesion and roughness of biomaterials through PM-EDM: a comprehensive review. *Materials and Manufacturing Processes*, 2020. 35(11): p. 1157–1180.

[16] Al-Amin, M., et al., Assessment of PM-EDM cycle factors influence on machining responses and surface properties of biomaterials: a comprehensive review. *Precision Engineering*, 2020. 66: p. 531–549.

[17] Aliyu, A.A.A., et al., A review of additive mixed-electric discharge machining: current status and future perspectives for surface modification of biomedical implants. *Advances in Materials Science and Engineering*, 2017. 2017, p. 1–23.

[18] Aliyu, A.A.A., et al. Synthesis and characterization of bioceramic oxide coating on Zr-Ti-Cu-Ni-Be BMG by electro discharge process. In *International Scientific-Technical Conference Manufacturing*. 2019. Springer, Germany.

[19] Aliyu, A.A.A., et al., Hydroxyapatite mixed-electro discharge formation of bioceramic Lakargiite (CaZrO3) on Zr–Cu–Ni–Ti–Be for orthopedic application. *Materials and Manufacturing Processes*, 2018. 33(16): p. 1734–1744.

[20] Prakash, C. and M.S. Uddin, Surface modification of β-phase Ti implant by hydroaxyapatite mixed electric discharge machining to enhance the corrosion resistance and in-vitro bioactivity. *Surface and Coatings Technology*, 2017. 326(Part A): p. 134–145.

[21] Prakash, C., et al. On the influence of nanoporous layer fabricated by PMEDM on β-Ti implant: biological and computational evaluation of bone-implant interface. in 5th International Conference of Materials Processing and Characterization, Hyderabad. 2016.

[22] Prakash, C., Kansal, H.K., Pabla, B.S. & Puri, S., Experimental investigations in powder mixed electric discharge machining of Ti-35Nb-7Ta-5Zr β-titanium alloy. *Materials and Manufacturing Processes*, 2016. 32(3), 274–285. doi:10.1080/10426914.2016.1198018.

[23] Oliveira, A.R.F., W.F. Sales, and A.A. Raslan, *Titanium perovskite (CaTiO3) formation in Ti6Al4V alloy using the electrical discharge machining process for biomedical applications*. Surface and Coatings Technology, the Netherlands.

[24] Rafique, M.M.A., Production and characterization of Zr based bulk metallic glass matrix composites (BMGMC) in the form of wedge shape ingots. *Engineering*, 2018. 10(04): p. 215.

[25] Hermawan, H., D. Ramdan, and J.R. Djuansjah, *Metals for Biomedical Applications*. 2011: INTECH Open Access Publisher, UK.

[26] Sales, W.F., A.R.F. Oliveira, and A.A. Raslan, Titanium perovskite (CaTiO3) formation in Ti6Al4V alloy using the electrical discharge machining process for biomedical applications. *Surface and Coatings Technology*, 2016. 307, Part A: p. 1011–1015.

5 Material Transfer Rate During Electro-Discharge Process
Modeling and Optimization

Abdul Azeez Abdu Aliyu, Ahmad Majdi Abdul-Rani, Iqtidar Ahmed Gul, Muhammad Usman, Boonrat Lohwongwatana, and Ahmad Nasiru Hamza

5.1 INTRODUCTION

The applications of electro-discharge machining (EDM) are advancing from tools and dies fabrication, to shaping of automobiles, aerospace, nuclear components and recently, to surface modification of biomedical implant [1]. Despite the complexity of the EDM process, several studies have revealed the wide potentialities of this process in the biomedical field, especially with regards to the fabrication and surface modification of metallic implant [1–5]. In recent years, EDM process have been hybridized by addition of powder particles into the dielectric fluid called powder mixed EDM (PM-EDM) [4, 6]. The chemical composition and surface chemistry of the substrate (workpiece) material is modified when a significant material from the suspended dielectric additives and tool-electrode are transferred to the workpiece surface [7, 8]. This serves as a strong route of providing a well finished and qualitative machined surface. In addition to generation of extremely hard, nano-finished, and non-porous surface, PM-EDM produces a bioactive and a biocompatible layer on the implant surface through the concept of material migration, especially when proper dielectric additives/tool-electrode combination is used [9, 10]. Batish et al. [11] investigated the mechanism of material transfer during EDM of three different die steel samples. Thus, confirmed a reasonable transfer of tool-electrode material and powder particles on the EDMed surface. Gülcan et al. [12] reported a substantial transfer of tool-electrode materials on the workpiece-electrode surface after PM-EDM. A very hard surface with strong abrasion and corrosion resistance layer was achieved. It is believed that, material transfer by PM-EDM altered the chemical content, mechanical properties as well as the metallurgical structure of the machined surface, thereby, forming different layers on the PM-EDMed surface [13]. The topmost layer is recast layer, which is produced because of re-solidification of unflushed metallic debris in the craters. The

DOI: 10.1201/9781003456018-5

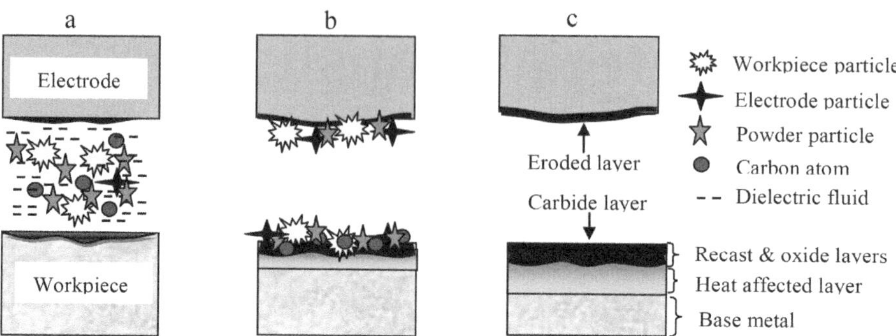

FIGURE 5.1 Mechanism of material migration and transfer. (a) Initiation of spark. (b) Carbon atoms, powder, and tool-electrode particles adhered on the electrodes surfaces. (c) Formation of three distinct layers.

hard carbide and oxide film constituted the middle layers. The carbide layer is formed due to the reaction of carbon in the hydrocarbon-based dielectric fluid or dielectric fluid additives and the workpiece alloying elements [7, 10]. On the other hand, a biocompatible oxide layer is developed due to fusion of oxygen (in the dielectric additives) and the elemental constituents in the workpiece material. The last layer is the heat affected zone (heated but non-melted layer). This layer is formed due to heating and subsequent quenching during the PM-EDM process. The characteristics of these layers mainly depend on the type of electrode material, dielectric fluid, and its additives as well as the setting of the input parameters [14]. The schematic illustration of material migration mechanism and material transfer during PM-EDM is displayed in Figure 5.1. In the first stage, a spark is generated through a powder suspended dielectric fluid. In this phase, the electrode materials are eroded, forming a large crater (Figure 1a). The detached electrodes particles, powder particles, and the carbon atoms migrated to the electrodes surfaces as shown in Figure 1b. The final stage is shown in Figure 1c, whereby all layers are completely formed with no or shallow craters on the PM-EDMed surface. However, the tool-electrode size reduced due to erosion of the contact surface.

Although, numerous studies have been reported with regards to PM-EDM, few researches could be found on the prediction of material transfer during PM-EDM process. This study attempt to estimate the material transfer rate (MTR) when EDM of Zr-based BMG by mixing hydroxyapatite powder to the dielectric fluid. The optimum parameters setting for maximizing the MTR to 0.007411 g/min is achieved. The predicted error of MTR was found to be 4.94%.

5.2 EXPERIMENTATION

The experiments of this study were planned and analyzed using Design Expert 10.0 software. FP60EA Mitsubishi die-sinker EDM machine was employed to machine the surface of the Zr-based BMG substrate. Prior to experiment, the weight of both

TABLE 5.1
Experimental conditions

Conditions	Unit	Descriptions
Gap voltage	V	12
Off-time (Toff)	μs	16
Workpiece	-	Zr-based BMG
Electrode (tool) type	-	Commercial pure titanium (CpTi)
Dielectric type	-	Hydrocarbon oil
Powder type	-	Hydroxyapatite (HA)
Machining depth	mm	0.3 mm
Flushing type	-	Emission
Discharge current	A	4, 8, 12
Discharge time	μs	4, 8, 16
Powder concentration	g/L	5, 10, 15, 20

the tool-electrode and workpiece specimens were recorded. The MTR of each treated sample is calculated by taking the difference between the weight of the specimen before and after the experiment divided by the machining time, same way as done by Watane and Gudadhe [15]. The influence of various process parameters on the MTR was analyzed using design expert 10.0 software. Response surface methodology using D-optimal design is a form of RSM was employed to plan, analyze, and optimize the MTR. In the current study, the four factors (Dc, Dt, Pc, and Ep) selected based on the screening experiment were used to generate empirical models and optimize the responses (MTR). The experimental conditions are summarized in Table 5.1.

5.3   RESULTS AND DISCUSSIONS

The ANOVA table indicating the contribution of each factor on the MTR is presented in Table 5.2. The "Prob>F" value of 0.0001 signifies that the model is significant. The table also shows that the factors Dc, Dt, Pc, Ep, and interactions AB, AD, BC, CD, and B^2 are significant model terms with "Prob>F" values <0.05. The lack-of-fit "Prob>F" value of 0.2170 indicates its insignificance relative to the pure error. Insignificant lack-of-fit is good, the model is required to fit the response (MTR).

The normal probability plot of the residuals plot shows that most of the data lie along the straight line as seen in Figure 5.2a. This confirmed that the selected terms are only the significant factors and the errors are normally distributed as noticed in Figure 5.2b. The residuals versus predicted values plot shows a randomly distributed data without any clear pattern as required. In the residuals versus run plot presented in Figure 5.2c, all the studentized residuals of regression lies within the required limit (±3 sigma), and no any outlier observed. This confirms the capability of the model to predict the MTR.

TABLE 5.2
ANOVA for quadratic model of the material transfer rate

Source	Sum of Squares	df	Mean Square	F Value	p-value Prob > F	
Model	17.82	13	1.37	26.35	<0.0001	**Significant**
A-Dc	0.39	1	0.39	7.52	0.0208	
B-Dt	0.42	1	0.42	8.15	0.0171	
C-Pc	6.24	1	6.24	119.9	<0.0001	
D-Ep	1.67	1	1.67	32.17	0.0002	
AB	1.49	1	1.49	28.67	0.0003	
AC	0.066	1	0.066	1.26	0.2875	
AD	0.35	1	0.35	6.81	0.0261	
BC	2.56	1	2.56	49.15	<0.0001	
BD	0.082	1	0.082	1.57	0.2383	
CD	1.07	1	1.07	20.58	0.0011	
A2	0.086	1	0.086	1.65	0.2286	
B2	1.38	1	1.38	26.51	0.0004	
C2	0.055	1	0.055	1.06	0.3268	
Residual	0.52	10	0.052			
Lack-of-fit	0.35	5	0.071	2.1	0.217	**Not significant**
Pure error	0.17	5	0.034			
Cor total	18.34	23				

Figure 5.3 shows the Box-Cox plot for power transformation of MTR. It could be observed that the confidence intervals (CIs) are between -0.45 and 0.1. The current position of the lambda is at 0, and the best position suggested by the software is -0.18. Therefore, the software recommended to use a log transformation to bring the lambda back to 0. However, in the current analysis, the difference is not that much, and the lambda is within the range of the CI. Therefore, the adopted transformation is good, changing to the software recommendation might resulted to some analysis problem such as loss of the model significance.

Figure 5.4 shows a one-factor effect plot for MTR. It could be noticed that the MTR is maintained constantly up to 8 A, and then slightly decreases with an increase in the Dc (Figure 5.4a). However, it increases with increase in Dt up to 10 μs and decreases with further increase in Dt (Figure 5.4b). Increase in both Dc and Dt resulted in a raise in discharge energy and hence more material erosion from both electrodes which resulted in high MTR. Beyond the current of 8 A and discharge time of 10 μs, MTR decreases, due to much higher energy which increases the machining gap and hence, sufficient gap flushing and less material transfer. Contentious raise in MTR was noticed when the HA concentration increased (Figure 5.4c). This is obvious that the addition of HA resulted in more concentration and hence higher material transfer. On the other hand, higher MTR is observed when positive tool-electrode polarity

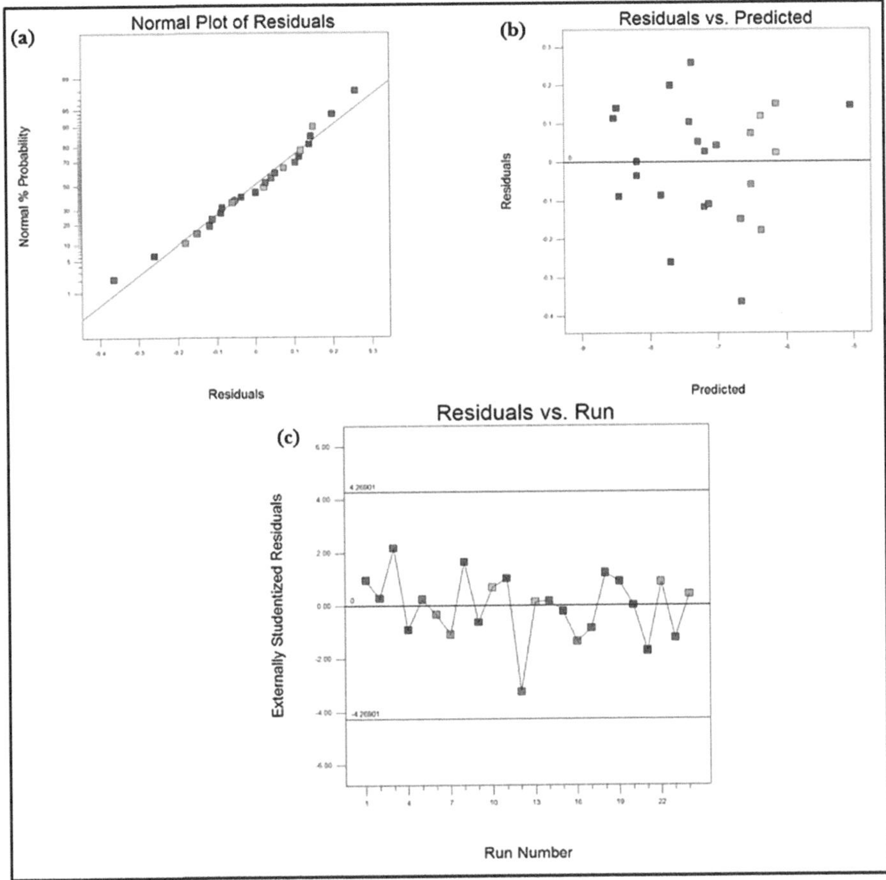

FIGURE 5.2 Residuals plots (a) normal plot (b) Residuals versus predicted (c) Residuals versus runs.

is used (Figure 5.4d). This might be due to higher tool-electrode wear observed in positive polarity setting compared to negative setting, which resulted in more tool-electrode material transfer on the substrate surface. The contours plots of the MTR are presented in Figure 5.5. The two-dimensional contour plots shown in Figure 5.5a–c indicate the MTR values in the contours.

A curved plot is observed in 3D surface plots presented in Figure 5.6a–c, which indicates the significance of the curvature and a quadratic model. The highest MTR is observed at 10 A and 8 μs parameters setting in the current versus discharge time 3D surface plot shown in Figure 5.6a. Moreover, the Pc versus Dc plot shows highest MTR of 0.002 g/min at Pc of 20 g/L and Dc of 5 A as observed Figure 5.6b. A similar MTR is achieved when Pc of 20 g/L and Dt of 8 μs parameters setting is employed as shown in Figure 6c.

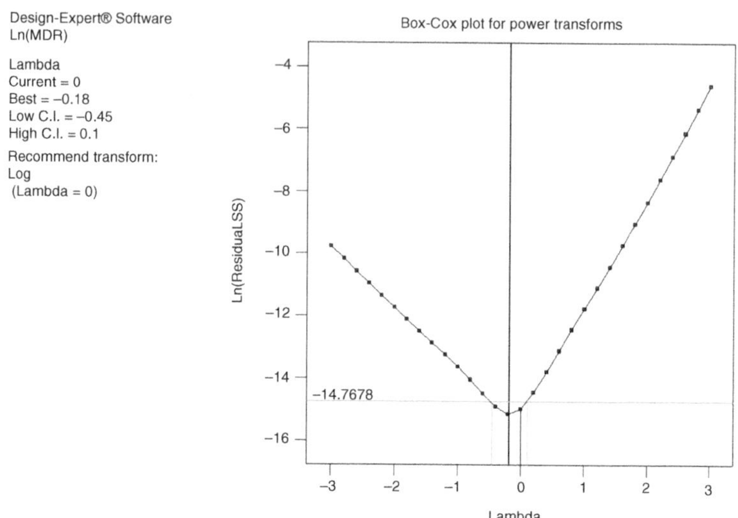

FIGURE 5.3　Box-Cox for power transformation of MTR.

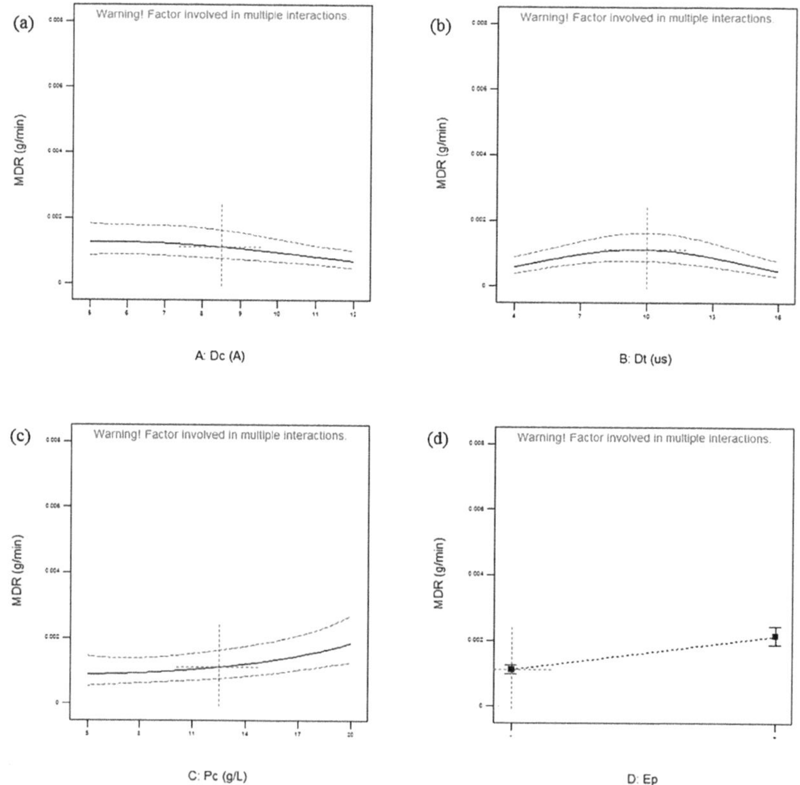

FIGURE 5.4　One factor effect plot for MTR. (a) Influence of Dc on MTR. (b) Influence of Dt on MTR. (c) Influence of Pc on MTR. (d) Influence of Ep on MTR.

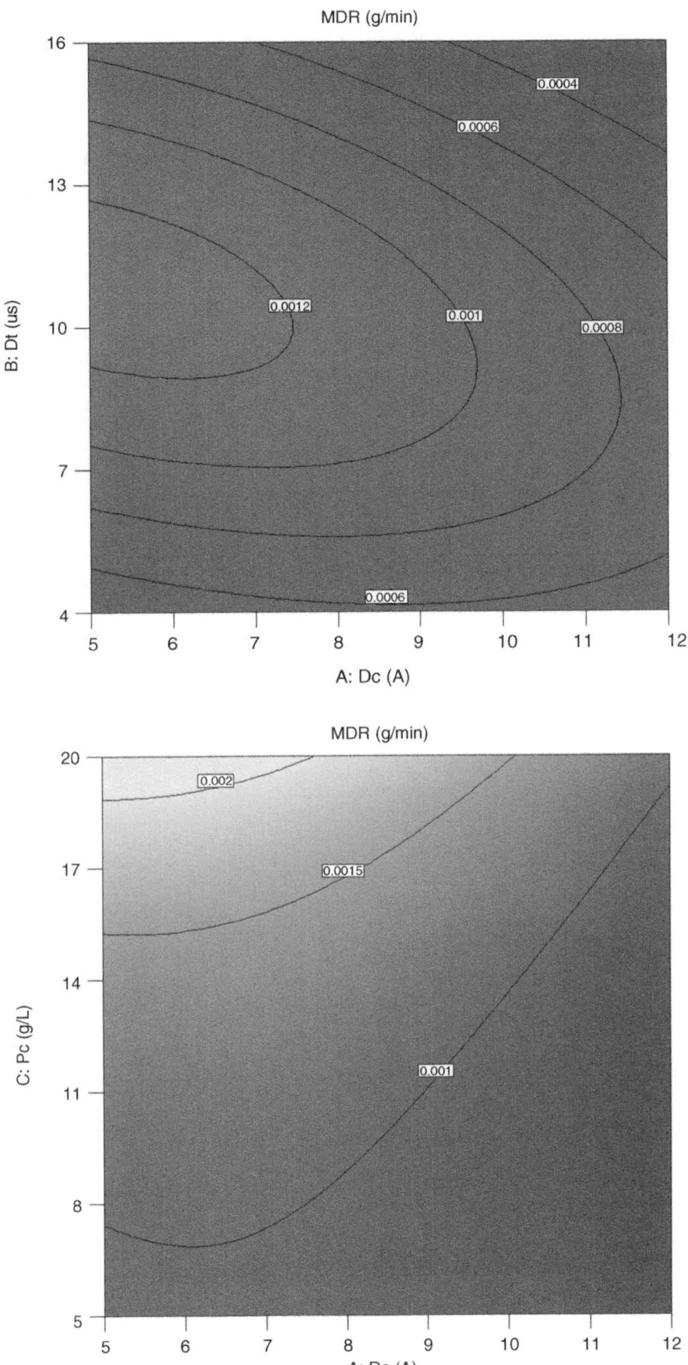

FIGURE 5.5 Contour plots showing the influence of Dc, Dt, and Pc process parameters on the MTR. (a) Dc versus Dt. (b) Pc versus Dc. (c) Pc versus Dt.

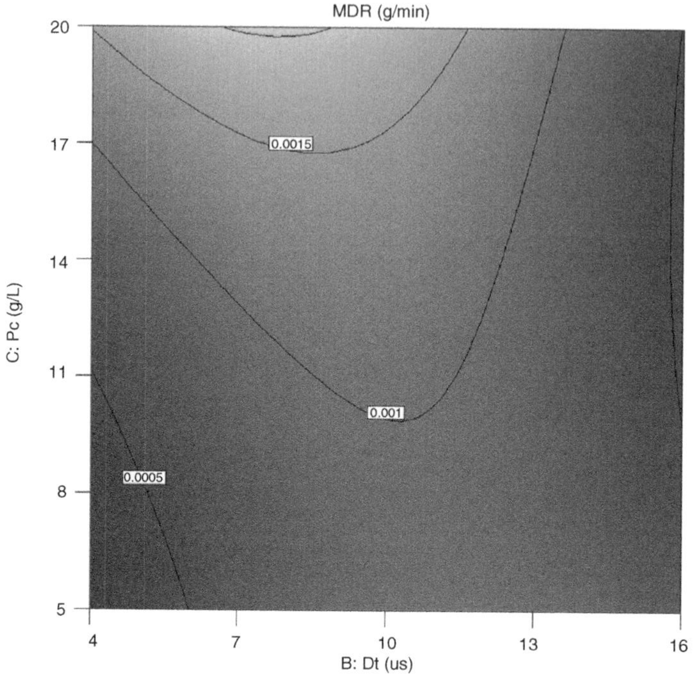

FIGURE 5.5 (Continued)

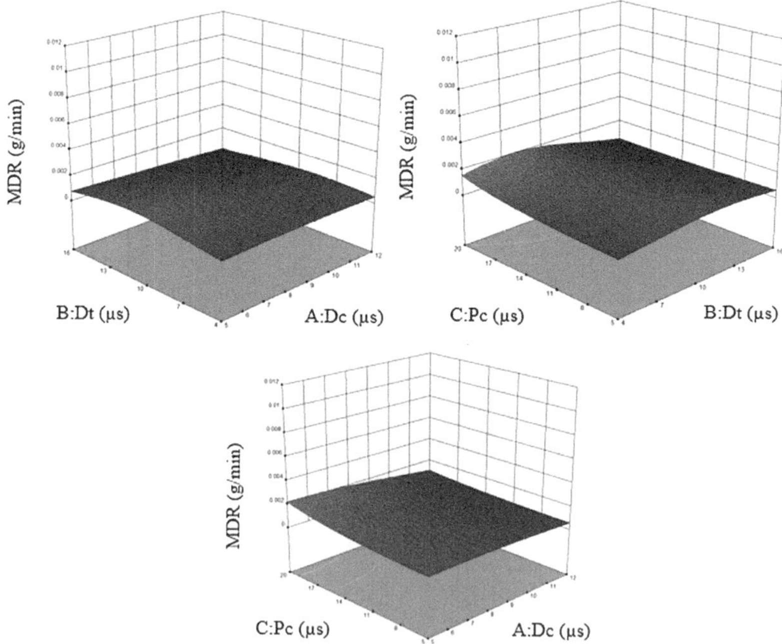

FIGURE 5.6 Three-dimensional surface plots for MTR. (a) Dt versus Dc. (b) Pc versus Dc. (c) Pc versus Dt.

5.3.1 Modeling of MTR

The ANOVA tables presented produces the equations which relate the response MTR and the input parameters. The final predicted model equations in terms of the actual factors for the MTR are presented in equation (5.1).

$$Ln(MTR) = -12.96631 + 0.44302 * Dc + 0.64098 * Dt + 0.18750 * Pc$$

$$-0.16032 * Dc*Dt - 2.56623E\text{-}003 * Dc*Pc - 0.010376$$

$$*Dt*Pc - 0.014847 * Dc^2 - 0.020995 * Dt^2 + 2.47001E\text{-}003 * Pc^2 \ldots \ldots \ldots .(5.1)$$

5.3.2 Model Adequacy for MTR

Table 5.3 shows the model summary statistic for MTR. The software recommended a quadratic model for the MTR, due to its least standard deviation (0.23), largest statistic R-square (0.7710), and lowest PRESS (4.20) compared to the linear model.

5.3.3 Optimization of MTR

The response optimization can be directly obtained from the design expert software by considering the response value and desirability. The software suggests the optimum parameters combination.

Maximizing Material Transfer Rate
Table 5.4 provides the constraints in design space while Table 5.5 gives the solutions suggested by the software for maximizing the MTR.

5.3.4 Confirmation Test

Following a successful selection of the input parameters' optimum level, a confirmation test was carried out to validate the models developed for the selected response (MTR). In this study, a confirmation test was conducted using the optimum parameters suggested by the design software. Thus, it will be possible to verify the adequacy of the developed mathematical models. Optimum parameters setting plays a significant

TABLE 5.3
Model summary statistic for MTR

Source	Std. Dev.	R-squared	Adjusted R-squared	Predicted R-squared	PRESS	
Linear	0.64	0.5788	0.4901	0.2712	13.37	
2FI	0.39	0.8918	0.8085	0.5517	8.22	
Quadratic	0.23	0.9716	0.9348	0.771	4.2	**Suggested**
Cubic	0.18	0.9909	0.9579		+	Aliased

TABLE 5.4
Constraints for maximizing MTR

Constraints

Name	Goal	Lower Limit	Upper Limit	Lower Weight	Upper Weight	Importance
A:Dc	Is in range	5	12	1	1	3
B:Dt	Is in range	4	16	1	1	3
C:Pc	Is in range	5	20	1	1	3
D:Ep	Is in range	-	+	1	1	3
MTR	**Maximize**	0.00019	0.0075	1	1	3

TABLE 5.5
Solutions for maximizing MTR suggested by the software

Number	Dc	Dt	Pc	Ep	MTR	Desirability	
1	9.081	7.227	19.973	±	0.008	1	**Selected**
2	9.302	6.492	19.996	+	0.008	1	
3	10.415	6.703	19.997	+	0.008	1	
4	10.261	5.904	20	+	0.008	1	
5	9.705	6.963	19.953	+	0.008	1	
6	10.032	6.766	19.974	+	0.008	1	
7	9.156	6.32	19.991	+	0.008	1	
8	9.443	6.686	19.949	+	0.008	1	
9	8.598	6.892	19.999	+	0.008	1	
10	9.886	6.647	19.943	+	0.008	1	
11	9.827	6.414	19.945	+	0.008	1	
12	8.924	7.06	19.985	+	0.008	1	
13	9.78	6.816	19.951	+	0.008	1	
14	9.418	7.27	19.993	+	0.008	1	
15	10.559	6.535	19.998	+	0.007	1	

role not only in improving the quality but also in the industries by reducing parts production time and cost. This study planned to achieve a minimum surface roughness for a nanostructured surface while maximizing the rate of material transfer. Four different tests of confirmation tests need to be conducted. The optimum parameters conditions are suggested by the design software and presented in Figures 5.7 and 5.8 as denoted by the red circle. These automated settings will be adopted in this study for conducting confirmation runs, and the MTR indicated by a blue circle in each figure, will be considered.

Table 5.6 displays the desirability and the CI of 95% of MTR. The CI results show that standard error of process parameters for MTR is within limits, i.e., around 5%.

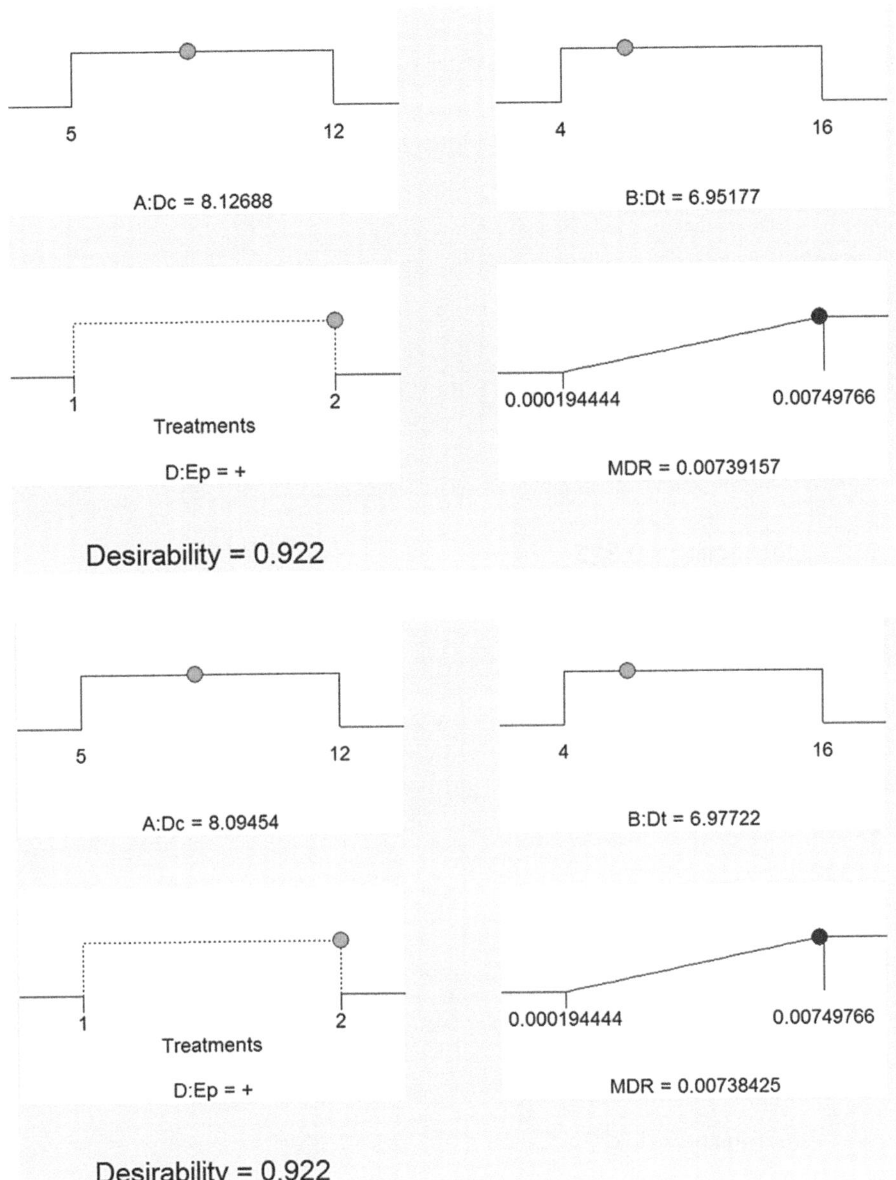

FIGURE 5.7 Optimized parameters settings 1 and 2.

Figure 5.9 gives the two-dimensional desirability and contour plots for the predicted MTR. Based on the design software, the desirability of the Dt and Dc parameters occurred at 0.922 when Dt = 8 μs and Dc = 8 A as depicted in Figure 5.9a. To achieve the highest MTR of 0.007389 g/min (Figure 5.9b), the desirable values of Dt = 8 μs and Dc = 8 A have to be adopted.

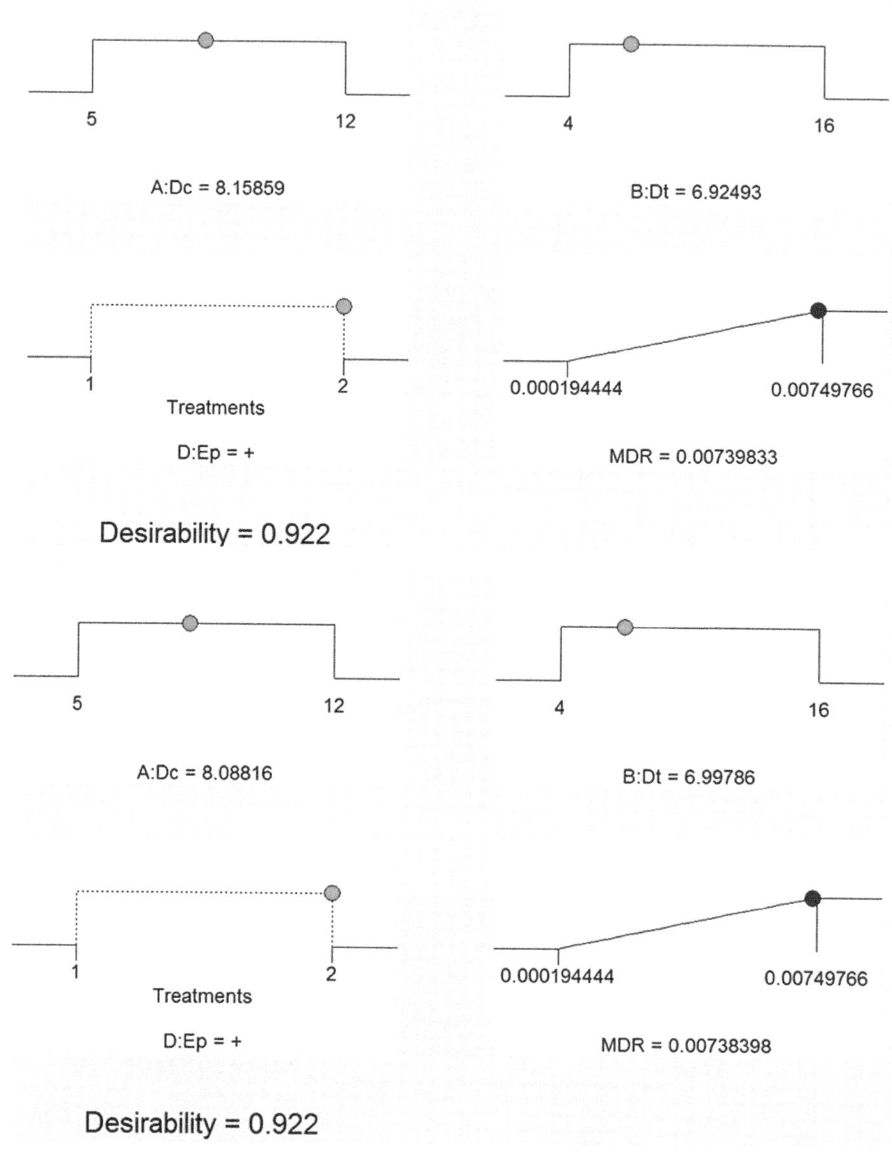

FIGURE 5.8 Optimized parameters settings 3 and 4.

Using the optimum parameters conditions generated by the software, five sets of confirmation test were carried out. The results of both responses are presented in Table 5.7. The five sets of results for the MTR provided by the software (predicated) and those conducted at optimum parameters setting (actual experiment) were compared in Table 5.8.

TABLE 5.6
Desirability and percentage confidence interval

Factor	Name	Level	Low level	High level	Std. Dev.	coding
A	Dc	8.12	5.00	12.00	0.00	Actual
B	Dt	6.95	4.00	16.00	0.00	Actual
C	Pc	20.00	5.00	20.00	0.00	Actual
D	Ep	+	-	+	N/A	Actual

Response	Predicted mean	Predicted median	Observed	Std. Dev.	SE mean	CI for mean		99% of population	
						95% CI low	95% CI high	95% Ti low	95% Ti high
MTR^2	0.007390	0.007202	-	0.0016	N/A	0.01258	0.808367	0.001817	0.028546

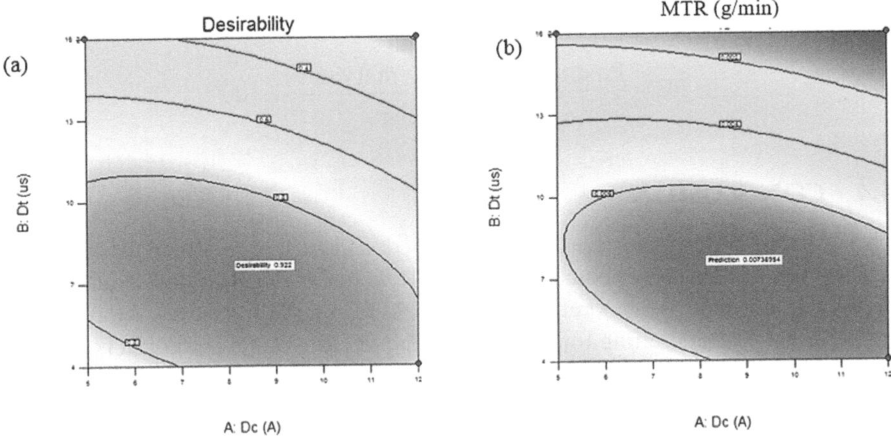

FIGURE 5.9 Two-dimensional contour plots for the desirability and the predicted values of the MTR. (a) Desirability value of Dt and Dc. (b) Desirability of Dt and Dc on MTR.

TABLE 5.7
Confirmation test results at optimized input parameters

Run order	Dc (A)	Dt (μs)	Ep	Pc (g/L)	MTR (g/min)
1	8.0	7.0	+	20	0.00693
2	8.0	7.0	+	20	0.00701
3	8.0	7.0	+	20	0.00712
4	8.0	7.0	+	20	0.00718
5	8.0	7.0	+	20	0.00687

TABLE 5.8
Result comparison for MTR

Run order	Experimental MTR (g/min)	Predicated MTR (g/min)	Percentage error (%)
1	0.00693	0.00739	5.82
2	0.00701	0.00738	5.01
3	0.00712	0.00740	3.78
4	0.00718	0.00739	2.84
5	0.00687	0.00741	7.29
Average predicted error		**4.94**	

To enable accuracy estimation of the predicted models, prediction error (PE) of the MTR was determined. The average error of the five results was also calculated to achieve the average PE (APE). The PE is calculated through equation (5.2). The APE for MTR was found to be 4.94. A predicted error less than 10% confirmed the excellent reproducibility of the experimental conclusions [16, 17].

$$PE = \frac{\text{Predicted} - \text{experimental values}}{\text{predicted value}} \times 100\% \tag{5.2}$$

5.4 CONCLUSION

The Zr-based BMG was successfully machined, and surface modified using the PM-EDM process. The model equations for MTR were developed. These equations can be used to estimate the theoretical values of MTR by the industries. Moreover, the optimum parameters setting for maximizing the MTR to 0.007411 g/min is achieved. The predicted error of MTR was found to be 4.94%. Based on the literature, the error was considered within the acceptable limit.

ACKNOWLEDGMENTS

The authors appreciated the financial support by UP-UTP international collaborative research fund with cost centers 015ME0-081 and 015LB0-040 for supporting this research.

REFERENCES

[1] A. A. A. Aliyu *et al.*, "A review of additive mixed-electric discharge machining: current status and future perspectives for surface modification of biomedical implants," *Advances in Materials Science and Engineering,* vol. 2017, 2017.

[2] M. Al-Amin, A. M. Abdul Rani, A. A. Abdu Aliyu, M. G. Bryant, M. Danish, and A. Ahmad, "Bio-ceramic coatings adhesion and roughness of biomaterials through PM-EDM: A comprehensive review," *Materials and Manufacturing Processes,* vol. 35, no. 11, pp. 1157–1180, 2020.

[3] M. Al-Amin *et al.*, "Assessment of PM-EDM cycle factors influence on machining responses and surface properties of biomaterials: A comprehensive review," *Precision Engineering,* vol. 66, pp. 531–549, 2020.

[4] M. Razak *et al.*, "The potential of improving the Mg-alloy surface quality using powder mixed EDM," in *Progress in Engineering Technology*: Springer, Germany, 2019, pp. 43–53.

[5] M. Razak, A. Rani, N. Saad, G. Littlefair, and A. Aliyu, "Controlling corrosion rate of magnesium alloy using powder mixed electrical discharge machining," in *IOP Conference Series: Materials Science and Engineering*, 2018, vol. 344, no. 1: IOP Publishing, Germany, p. 012010.

[6] M. Al-Amin, A. M. Abdul Rani, A. A. Abdu Aliyu, M. A. H. Abdul Razak, S. Hastuty, and M. G. Bryant, "Powder mixed-EDM for potential biomedical applications: A critical review," *Materials and Manufacturing Processes,* vol. 35, no. 16, pp. 1789–1811, 2020.

[7] A. Aliyu, A. Abdul-Rani, T. Ginta, C. Prakash, E. Axinte, and R. Fua-Nizan, "Fabrication of nanoporosities on metallic glass surface by hydroxyapatite mixed EDM for orthopedic application," in *Int Med Device Technol Conf*, 2017, pp. 168–171.

[8] E. Axinte, A. Bofu, Y. Wang, A. M. Abdul-Rani, and A. A. A. Aliyu, "An overview on the conventional and nonconventional methods for manufacturing the metallic glasses," in *MATEC Web of Conferences*, 2017, vol. 112: EDP Sciences, p. 03003.

[9] A. a. A. Aliyu *et al.*, "Hydroxyapatite electro discharge coating of Zr-based bulk metallic glass for potential orthopedic application," in *Key Engineering Materials*, 2019, vol. 796: Trans Tech Publ, pp. 123–128.

[10] A. A. A. Aliyu *et al.*, "Electro-discharge machining of Zr67Cu11Ni10Ti9Be3: An investigation on hydroxyapatite deposition and surface roughness," *Processes,* vol. 8, no. 6, p. 635, 2020.

[11] A. Batish, A. Bhattacharya, V. Singla, and G. Singh, "Study of material transfer mechanism in die steels using powder mixed electric discharge machining," *Materials and Manufacturing Processes,* vol. 27, no. 4, pp. 449–456, 2012.

[12] O. Gülcan, İ. Uslan, Y. Usta, and C. Çoğun, "Performance and surface alloying characteristics of Cu–Cr and Cu–Mo powder metal tool electrodes in electrical discharge machining," *Machining Science and Technology,* vol. 20, no. 4, pp. 523–546, 2016.

[13] J. Soni and G. Chakraverti, "Experimental investigation on migration of material during EDM of die steel (T215 Cr12)," *Journal of Materials Processing Technology,* vol. 56, no. 1–4, pp. 439–451, 1996.

[14] J.-P. Kruth, L. Stevens, L. Froyen, and B. Lauwers, "Study of the white layer of a surface machined by die-sinking electro-discharge machining," *CIRP Annals,* vol. 44, no. 1, pp. 169–172, 1995.

[15] K. H. Watane, "Enhancement of surface hardness of cutting tools by surface coating using EDM." *International Journal of Mechanical Engineering and Information Technology* 2(7), 614–630.

[16] H. Kansal, S. Singh, and P. Kumar, "Parametric optimization of powder mixed electrical discharge machining by response surface methodology," *Journal of Materials Processing Technology,* vol. 169, no. 3, pp. 427–436, 2005.

[17] M. J. Mir, K. Sheikh, B. Singh, and N. Malhotra, "Modeling and analysis of machining parameters for surface roughness in powder mixed EDM using RSM approach," *International Journal of Engineering, Science and Technology,* vol. 4, no. 3, pp. 45–52, 2012.

6 Arc Discharge Method for Aluminium Oxide Nanoparticle Synthesis

Shahruzaman Sulaiman, Ahmad Majdi Abdul-Rani, T V V L N Rao, Mohd Danish, and Maysarah Binti Al-Amin

6.1 INTRODUCTION AND BACKGROUND

For the past decades, metal nanoparticles development attracts numerous researchers around the world because of their novel physical, electrical, thermal, catalytic properties, and interdisciplinary applications [1]. The problem with current nanoparticle synthesis is high in cost hence, manufacturer need to create a cheaper process or material for the production nanoparticle materials [2]. The material proposed here is Aluminium 6061 by using arc discharge machine in pure water, without any chemical additives.

The next problem is the synthesizing method using available machine such as pulverized ball milling. Pulverized ball milling produces nanoparticles larger size than 100 nM [3]. The amount of nanoparticles produced is very limited and the evidence can be seen from the lower concentration of nanoparticles in aqueous state [4]. Hence to solve the problems, a preparation of aluminium oxide (Al_2O_3) nanoparticle via arc discharge machine using Aluminium 6061 material was prepared. Later, an analysis was made to observe the metallurgy of Al_2O_3 nanoparticle using SEM. Finally, the composition of aluminium nanoparticle was characterized using EDX spectroscopy.

6.2 ALUMINIUM OXIDE (AL$_2$O$_3$) NANOPARTICLES

Al_2O_3 nanoparticles attract attentions in selecting metal particles and widely used in variety areas such as medical, automotive industries, and biochemical [5]. Figure 6.1 illustrates the atomic structure of Al_2O_3.

A synthesis method developed involving wide variety of liquid and vapor reaction phase involving aluminium nanoparticles. These include wire explosion, laser ablation, combustion flame, and wet chemical process [6]. Few researchers studied the formation of alumina nanoparticles through aluminium droplet combustion.

DOI: 10.1201/9781003456018-6

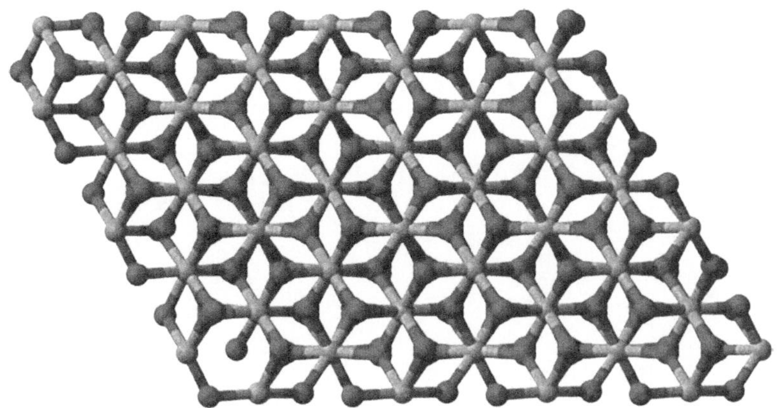

FIGURE 6.1 Crystal structure of aluminium oxide, α-Al_2O_3.

Researchers got to know that aluminium nanoparticles generated composed of primary particle in the size of 10–140 nm [7].

Other researchers use laser ablation technique on aluminium that was immersed in water and ethanol saturated with hydrogen [8]. They found that the shape of aluminium nanoparticle is almost spherical in shape with size range from 30 to 50 nm. Sindhu et al. [9] generate aluminium nanoparticle using wire explosion technique through different inert ambiences. The particles generated also have the mean dimeter size from 30nm to 45nm. Lee and Kim [10] prepared aluminium particles with geometric mean diameters of 139–614 nm and good monodispersity in dibutyl ether by a wet chemical process. They found that by using oleic acid as an organic surfactant to the precursor solution, the size of aluminium particles has reduced to approximately 35nm.

Sahu et al. [11] synthesized ethylene glycol-based alumina nanofluids through chemical routes. The average particle size was found to be 43 nm. Ghorbani [12] has used aerosol synthesis method to generate aluminium nanoparticles. The size of polyhedral aluminium particles lies in the range of 50–100 nm with an average particle size of approximately 87 nm.

6.3 METHOD TO PREPARE, ANALYZE, AND CHARACTERIZE ALUMINIUM OXIDE (AL$_2$O$_3$) NANOPARTICLE

To achieve the objective of this project, planning of the overall process must be in conjunction with the collection of data from explored research and experimental study. There are several steps that were planned before conducting this experiment. The experimental setup is explained in the next section.

The type of aluminium used was Al 6061 as shown in Figure 6.2. The diameter size of aluminium electrode is 5 mm with 200 mm in length. There are four bending points available in this electrode, bent at the angles of 90°. The dimension was already measured for each bending point. The electrode is then placed inside the beaker.

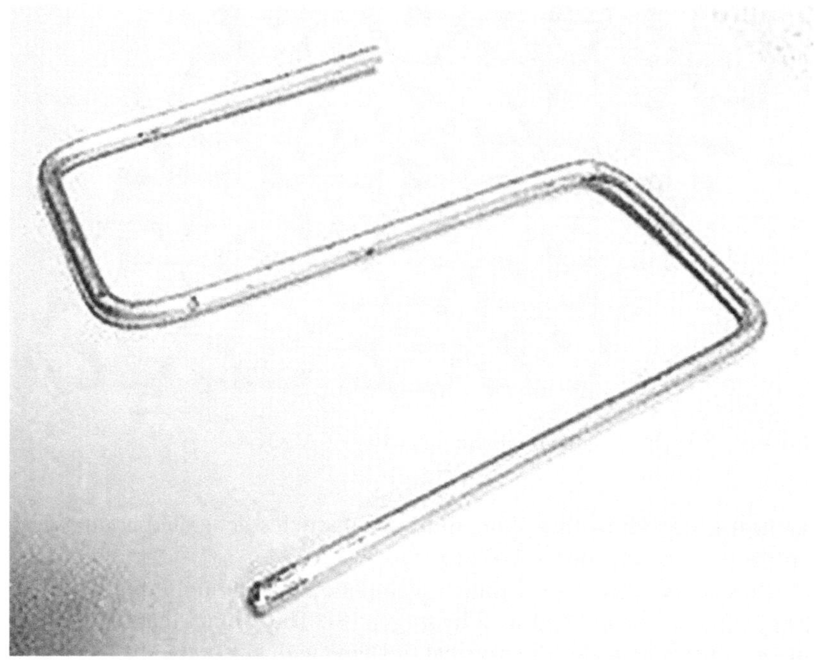

FIGURE 6.2   Diameter of 5 mm Al 6061 rod.

6.4 MACHINES AND APPARATUS SETUP

In this section, preparation of machine and apparatus is written. All arrangement and configuration are prepared in order to produce Al_2O_3 nanoparticle. The apparatus or machine are arc discharge machine, deionized water (DI water), adjustable DC programmable power supply, SEM, and EDX spectroscopy.

The complete system of arc discharge machine include integrated circuit and Arduino software were shown in Figure 6.3. The principle of the arc discharge machine is similar to electro-discharge machine (EDM).

6.5 DEIONIZED WATER

Figure 6.4 shows DI water which is used to fill in the beaker using arc discharge machine. The properties of the liquid are neutral (pH value 7) and electrolytic conductivity is 0.055 μS/cm. DI water is the most beneficial dielectric medium for preventing the oxidation of newly formed materials during the arc discharge process [13]. Without the positive charge of the oxidation layer, the colloid became highly unstable, and the composite particles will precipitate, and the Al_2O_3 nanoparticles settle out of the medium. The advantage of using pure water as dielectric medium

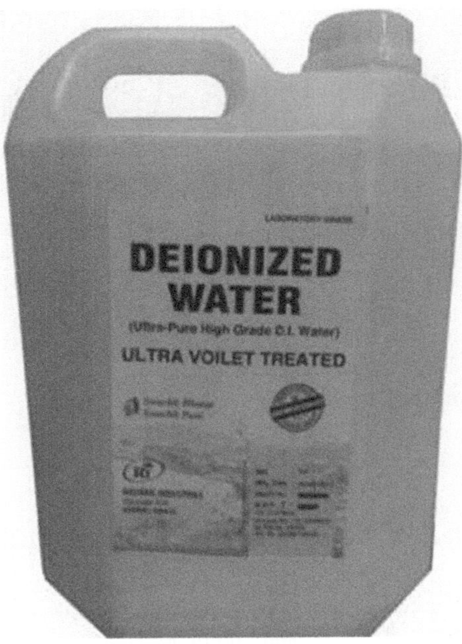

FIGURE 6.3   Complete system of arc discharge machine.

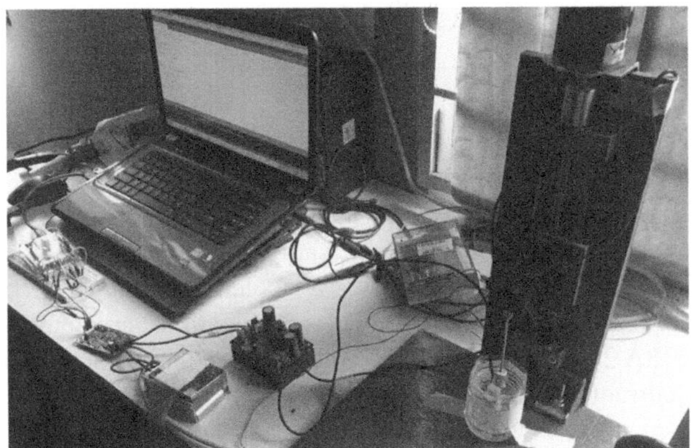

FIGURE 6.4   Deionized water 40 ml.

is the settled Al_2O_3 nanoparticles still can disperse again by using mechanically induced vibrations.

Figure 6.5 shows DC power supply. The maximum power for this power supply unit generated is up to 90 W, and maximum voltage produce is 30 voltages (V) with maximum currents of 3 A.

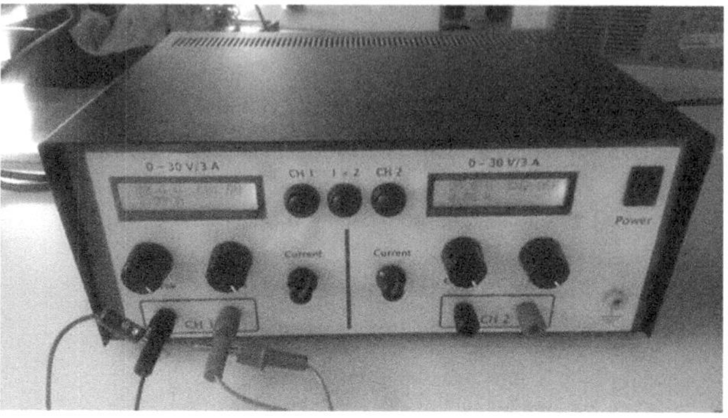

FIGURE 6.5   DC power supply.

TABLE 6.1
The parameters of the arc discharge process

Variable	Setup
Electrode	Aluminum 6061
Polarity	Positive and negative (EDM process)
Voltage (V)	18, 22, 26
Current (amp)	1, 2, 3
Temperature	Room temperature (25°C)
Duration	30 min
Dielectric fluid	Pure water

6.6   PARAMETER SETUP

The arc discharge machine setup is shown in Table 6.1. The voltage produced at each spark process were different. In this phase, samples need to be categorized according to parameter combinations. The samples are labeled according to parameters to differentiate the aluminium nanoparticle. The combination parameters are [1A 18V], [2A 22V], and [3A 26V] were tested. The investigated factors on this case are voltage and discharge current as shown in Table 6.1.

6.7   EXPERIMENT PROCEDURE ON SYNTHESIS OF AL$_2$O$_3$ NANOPARTICLES BY ARC DISCHARGE MACHINE

Figure 6.6 shows the flow chart that represents workflow of a process for Al$_2$O$_3$ nanoparticle synthetization production using arc discharge method. The material selected is Al 6061. The second phase is to determine of arc discharge parameters used for effective production. The parameters which were chosen are based on the combination of voltage and current to generate a spark when both electrodes touch

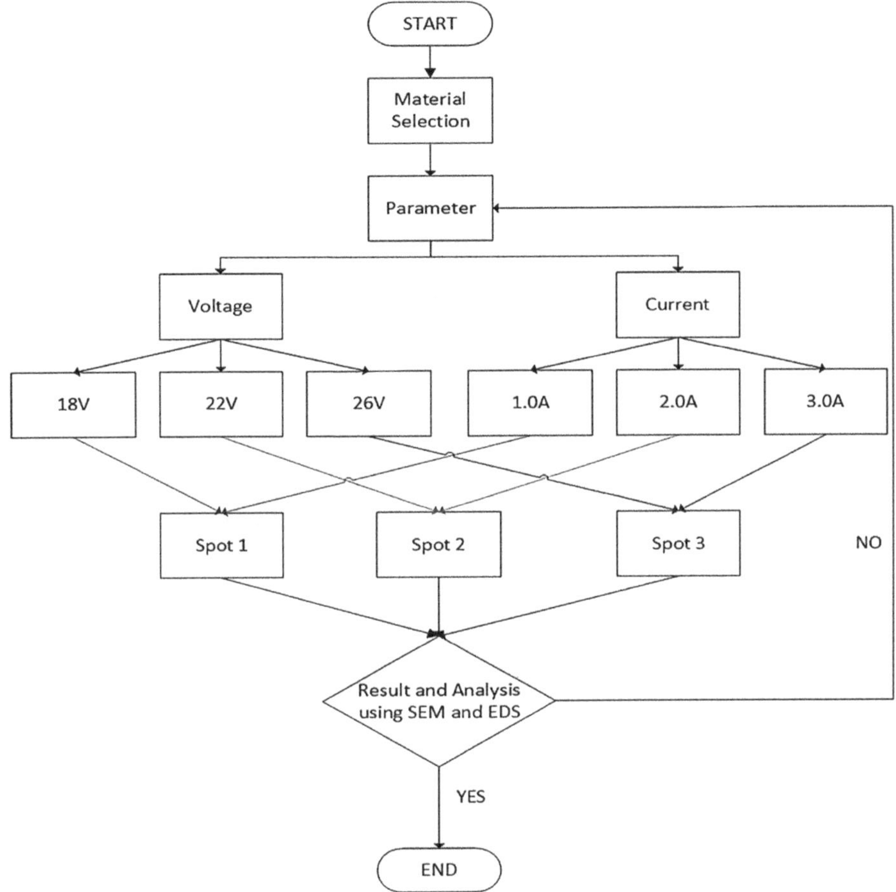

FIGURE 6.6 Overall process for Al_2O_3 nanoparticle synthesizing.

each other due to different polarity which is anode(+) and cathode(-). The third phase is to analyze the appearance and metallurgy of each spot using SEM and EDX. If the result obtained is not satisfactory, the experiment is calibrated again by adjusting the parameter phase. The last phase of this experiment is to bring the product Al_2O_3 powder and immerse it in the dielectric fluid.

The schematic diagram of the arc discharge machine is illustrated in Figure 6.7. The machine consists of a tool-electrode (cathode) and a workpiece-electrode (anode) separated by a small gap known as spark gap and submerged in a dielectric medium (DI water). The experiments were conducted using two aluminium electrodes (Al-6061), size Ø5 mm. The electrodes were located opposite to each other towards a vertical axis separated by a small gap and submerged in dielectric fluid (DI water). The gap and the value of voltage applied is associated with the temperature of dielectric

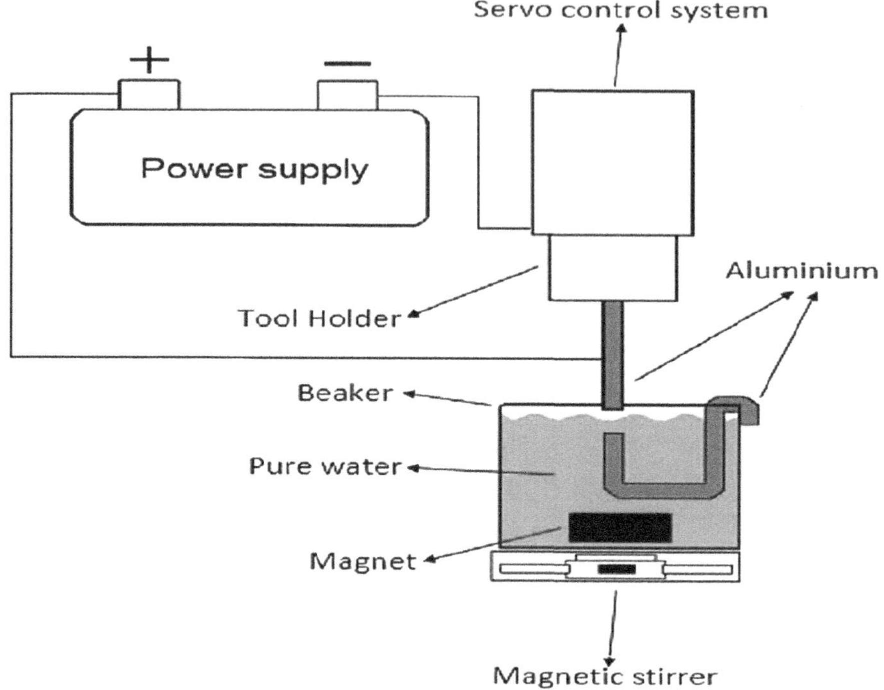

FIGURE 6.7   Illustration of arc discharge machining process.

fluid effect that occurs during the spark discharge between electrodes [14]. The movable cathode was located at top, while the fixed anode at the bottom.

Contacting the electrodes at the beginning of the process will produce the arc discharge as show in Figure 6.9 due to the various high-potential gradient across the electrodes, dielectric fluid breakdown occurs in the fluid and a plasma channel is formed [15]. This enables the discharge to take place though the dielectric fluid. Each spark discharge melts and suspends a small amount of material from the electrodes, and thus, a large particle part of the material is deposited at the base container [16]. The discharge device supplied a 18–26 V DC voltage and current value is 1–3.0 A. The volume of DI water had been fixed, which is 50 ml.

6.8   SEM ANALYSIS

The performance of Al_2O_3 nanoparticle is strongly related to the specific surface area. The size distribution of nanoparticles is a vital parameter especially for aluminium air battery application [17]. SEM can show the component breakdown of aluminium samples. Besides that, the specimen must be stroked by electron beam only on aluminium particles sample. The colloidal aluminium has been analyzed for the composition of aluminium nanoparticles. EDX analysis is used to analyze the differences in the composite makeup between the smaller and larger particle clusters [18]. This will explain the reason behind the production of bubbles during the synthesis of aluminium nanoparticles in a dielectric composed of DI water.

The analysis result of this research is to investigate the composition (wt%) and the physical appearance or metallurgy or also called SEM micrograph of the Al_2O_3 nanoparticles synthesis by the arc discharge process. Each spot is examined using SEM and EDX.

The SEM image reveal that the resultant aluminium nanoparticles are clearly non-uniform in terms of particle size. Comparison of the distance between the aluminium nanoparticles in the image reveals that the particles are well-dispersed overall, although the presence of some particle clustering can still be observed [19].

Other than that, SEM image analysis of the Al_2O_3 nanoparticle via the arc discharge machine shows an image of bulk solid composed of a large number of very fine particles. The shape is also called granular materials [20].

6.8.1 Experimental Result for Spot 1

Spot 1 is named due to parameter set used. The voltage selected for Spot 1 is 18 V and the current selected for aluminium nanoparticle synthesis is 1 A. Figure 6.8 shows that there are two emission peaks of aluminium and oxide at 1.40 and 0.48 keV. Those two peaks show that both aluminium (Al) and oxygen (O) show the highest value of substance composition contain in the sample. The sample aluminium particle at 18 V contain 35.02% elements of Al, and 52.52% elements of O. Transformed to equivalent atomic calculation (at%), whereby there are 23.43% elements of aluminium and 59.24% elements of oxide.

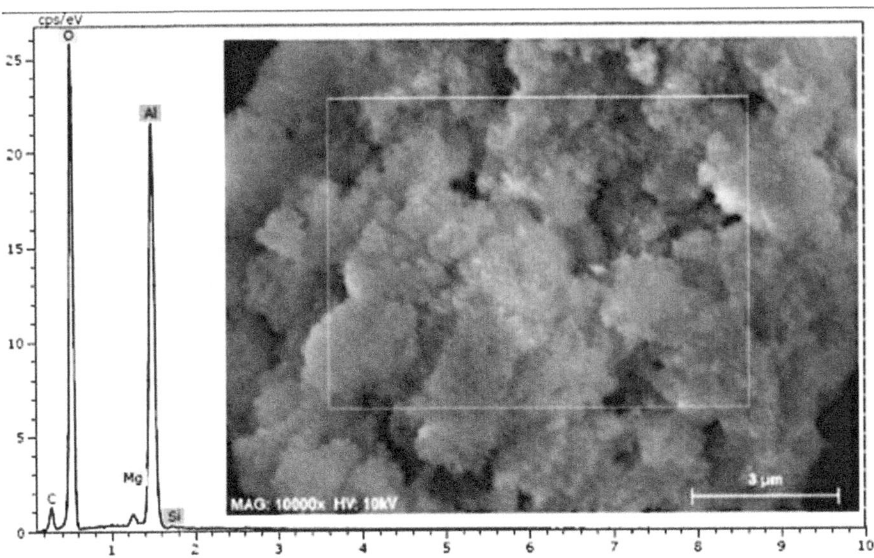

FIGURE 6.8 Illustration of aluminum metallurgy using SEM and EDX on Spot 1.

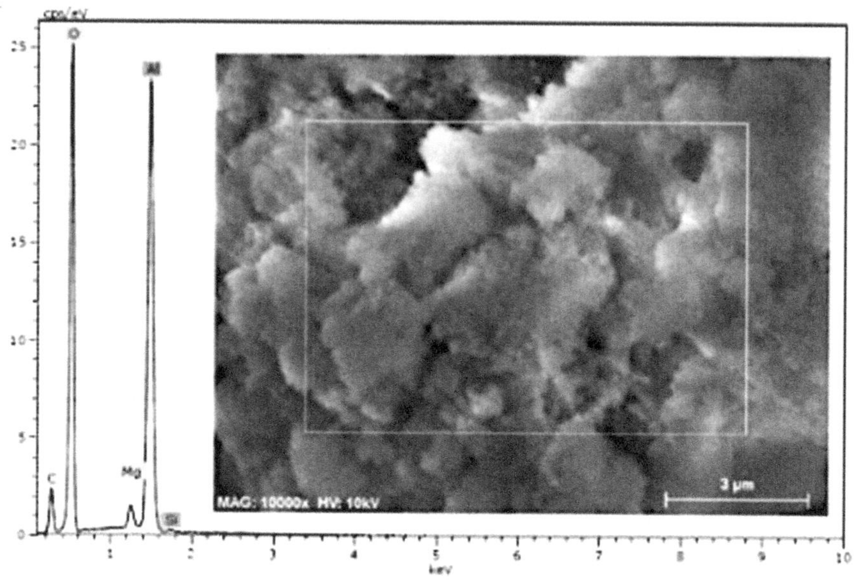

FIGURE 6.9　Illustration of aluminum metallurgy using SEM and EDX on Spot 2.

6.8.2　Experimental Result for Spot 2

Spot 2 is named due to parameter set used. The voltage selected for Spot 2 is 22 V and the current selected for aluminium nanoparticle synthesis is 2 A. Figure 6.9 shows that there are two emission peaks of aluminium and oxide at 1.38 and 0.46 keV. Those two peaks show that both aluminium (Al) and oxygen (O) show the highest value of substance composition contain in the sample. The sample aluminium particle at 22 V contain 35.07% elements of Al, and 56.71% elements of O. Transformed to equivalent atomic calculation (at%), whereby there are 23.72% elements of aluminium and 64.66% elements of oxide.

6.8.3　Experimental Result for Spot 3

Spot 3 is named due to parameter set used. The voltage selected for Spot 3 is 26 V and the current selected for aluminium nanoparticle synthesis is 3 A. Figure 6.10 shows that there are two emission peaks of aluminium and oxide at 1.36 and 0.45 keV. Those two peaks show that both aluminium (Al) and oxygen (O) show the highest value of substance composition contain in the sample. The sample aluminium particle at 26 V contain 36.20% elements of Al, and 56.48% elements of O. Transformed to equivalent atomic calculation (at%), whereby there are 24.70% elements of aluminium and 65.00% elements of oxide.

To summarize overall findings for three spots, comparison in terms of elements were made. The elements present during Al_2O_3 nanoparticle synthesizing are carbon, oxide, aluminium, magnesium, and silicone. Total composition weightage and atomic calculation are 100%. However, two main elements that are looked into

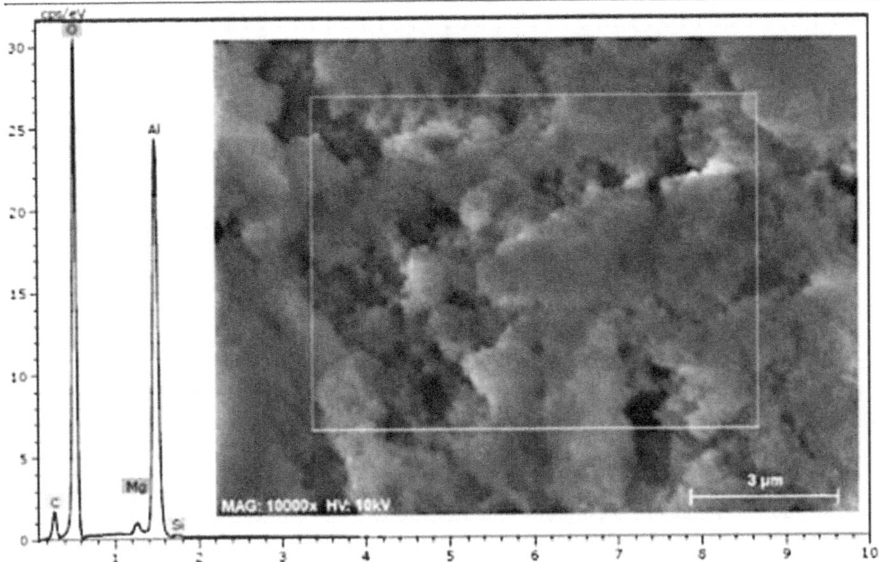

FIGURE 6.10   Illustration of aluminum metallurgy using SEM and EDX on Spot 3.

TABLE 6.2
Overall results for three spots produced by arc discharge machine

	Spot 1		Spot 2		Spot 3	
Elements	Composition weightage (%)	Atomic calculation (%)	Composition weightage (%)	Atomic calculation (%)	Composition weightage (%)	Atomic calculation (%)
C	10.67	16.03	7.12	10.82	6.16	9.45
O	52.52	59.24	56.71	64.66	56.48	65.00
Mg	1.54	1.15	0.90	0.67	0.93	0.71
Al	35.02	23.43	35.07	23.72	36.20	24.70
Si	0.24	0.16	0.20	0.13	0.23	0.15

are aluminium and oxide. Observe from Table 6.2, aluminium and oxide have relatively large amount presented. To simplify this table, higher the voltage and current supplied by arc discharge machine to aluminium, the greater the composition weightage produced.

The effect of different parameters on the morphology of product were studied by varying different parameter of DC voltage supply (18, 22, and 26 V) and average current (1, 2, and 3 A) repetitively. The reactions of synthesis and modification were performed at atmospheric, and all of the other parameters were held constant. After the arc discharge plasma process, Al_2O_3 could be found and collected from the three different sampling result as in Figure 6.8 in the container of dielectric liquid (DI water).

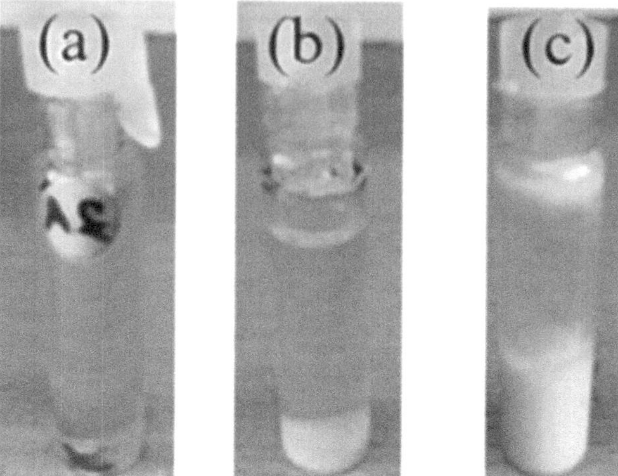

FIGURE 6.11   Images of aluminum oxide on three spots diluted in 10 ml deionized water solution.

As for the reasons, the Al_2O_3 nanoparticle was evaporated at increasing temperature and would condense into viscous liquid droplets during arc discharge process [21]. According to typical reference, the material removal mechanism in plasma arc discharge is associated with the thermal erosive effect that occurs during the spark discharge between two electrodes [22]. Due to a very high potential gradient across the two electrodes, dielectric fluid breakdown occurs in the fluid and a plasma channel is formed [23]. The enables the discharge to take place through the dielectric fluid. Every spark discharge melt and evaporates a small amount of material from both the electrodes and thus, a part of molten material is removed from the inter-electrode leaving a small carter on both the electrodes [24].

Figure 6.11 represents photographs of three samples of Al_2O_3 nanoparticle dispersed in DI water after running the arc discharge process for 30 min in 50ml of DI water. Because of hydrophobic property, aluminium oxide nanoparticle was hardly dissolved in water as shown in Figure 6.11a. It was noted that treated Al_2O_3 nanoparticle at 18 V began to disperse in DI water though they also formed largest aggregates and precipitate. Figure 6.11b and c shows the Al_2O_3 nanoparticle treated at 22 and 26 V, respectively. These results clearly demonstrate that the Al_2O_3 nanoparticle was generated via portable arc discharge and was proven in the result.

6.9 CONCLUSIONS

This research uses the arc discharge machine, developed by the combination of micro-electromechanical control and mechanical construction design, to produce Al_2O_3 nanoparticles. Using plasma system with arc discharge method as theoretical foundation, smaller and more evenly qualified aluminium nanoparticles are synthesized.

The properties of the produced Al_2O_3 nanoparticles have been identified by the SEM and EDX. From the experimental results, the primary advantage of using the plasma arch discharge system in Al_2O_3 nanoparticle synthesis is that the desired metallic materials are directly synthesized within the dielectric, could rapidly cool down the re-solidification of newly formed synthesized nanoparticles. The natural dispersion of nanoparticles directly synthesized within the dielectric medium, may avoid aggregation into large particles during collection process [25]. In this study, arc discharge machine could produce aluminium nanoparticles reaching average particle size diameter ranging from 20 to 30 nm.

When plasma arch discharge system uses pure water as aluminium nanoparticles, the newly formed of aluminium nanoparticles were being oxidized by water to produce Al_2O_3 nanoparticles. An oxidation layer on the surface of the particles causes particles to mutually repulse and prevents particles from aggregating or precipitating [26]. Thus, Al_2O_3 nanoparticles can remain as a suspension in pure water for an extended period of time at room temperature.

As its activity greatly increases, oxidation of Al_2O_3 nanoparticles was easily achieved. With the Al_2O_3 nanoparticle enabling to prevent its internal oxidation by the surface oxidative layer alone, this reaction process could release huge amounts of hydrogen. This property of Al_2O_3 nanoparticles could be used in production, storage, or transport of hydrogen.

The arc discharge method is a cheap, effective, rapid, and reliable process for nanoparticle production. Furthermore, the arc discharge method could simplify the production of Al_2O_3 nanoparticles, which may benefit for nanotechnology industries in the future. Industrial use of the system has the advantage of producing large quantities of colloidal metals at low cost compared to traditional means.

REFERENCES

[1] Sharma, G., Kumar, A., Sharma, S., Naushad, M., Prakash Dwivedi, R., ALOthman, Z. A., & Mola, G. T. (2017). Novel development of nanoparticles to bimetallic nanoparticles and their composites: A review. *Journal of King Saud University – Science,* 31 (2), 257–269. doi:10.1016/j.jksus.2017.06.012.

[2] Charitidis, C. A., Georgiou, P., Koklioti, M. A., Trompeta, A.-F., & Markakis, V. (2014). Manufacturing nanomaterials: from research to industry. *Manufacturing Review, 1, 11.*

[3] Paul, K. T., Satpathy, S. K., Manna, I., Chakraborty, K. K., & Nando, G. B. (2007). Preparation and characterization of nano structured materials from fly ash: A waste from thermal power stations, by high energy ball milling. *Nanoscale Research Letters, 2(8), 397–404.*

[4] Khan, I., Saeed, K., & Khan, I. (2017). Nanoparticles: Properties, applications and toxicities. *Arabian Journal of Chemistry, 12 (7), 908–931.* doi:10.1016/j.arabjc.2017.05.011.

[5] Yanık, F., & Vardar, F. (2015). Toxic effects of aluminum oxide (Al2O3) nanoparticles on root growth and development in *Triticum aestivum. Water, Air, & Soil Pollution, 226(9), 296.*

[6] Yanık, B., Ağustos, H., İpek, Y., Koyun, A., & Uzunsoy, D. (2013). Synthesis and characterization of aluminium nanoparticles by electric arc technique. *Arabian Journal for Science and Engineering, 38(12), 3587–3592.*

[7] Sahu, R. K., & Hiremath, S. S. (2017). Synthesis of aluminium nanoparticles in a water/ polyethylene glycol mixed solvent using μ-EDM. *IOP Conference Series: Materials Science and Engineering, 225, 012257.*

[8] Stratakis, E., Barberoglou, M., Fotakis, C., Viau, G., Garcia, C., & Shafeev, G. A. (2009). Generation of Al nanoparticles via ablation of bulk Al in liquids with short laser pulses. *Optics Express*, 17(15), 12650.

[9] T. K. Sindhu, R. Sarathi and S.R. Chakravarthy, "Generation and characterization of nano aluminium powder obtained through wire explosion process," *Bulletin of Materials Science*, vol. 30 (2), pp. 187–195, May 2014.

[10] Lee, H. M., & Kim, Y.-J. (2011). Preparation of size-controlled fine Al particles for application to rear electrode of Si solar cells. *Solar Energy Materials and Solar Cells*, 95(12), 3352–3358.

[11] Sahu, R. K., Hiremath, S. S., Manivannan, P. V., & Singaperumal, M. (2014). An innovative approach for generation of aluminium nanoparticles using micro electrical discharge machining. *Procedia Materials Science*, 5, 1205–1213.

[12] Ghorbani, H. (2014). A review of methods for synthesis of Al nanoparticles. *Oriental Journal of Chemistry*, 30(4), 1941–1949.

[13] J. Chandradass, D.-S, "Synthesis and characterization of alumina nanoparticles by Igepal CO-520 stabilized reverse micelle and sol-gel processing," *Materials and Manufacturing Processes*, 2015, vol. 23, pp. 494–498.

[14] Kolli, M., & Kumar, A. (2015). Effect of dielectric fluid with surfactant and graphite powder on electrical discharge machining of titanium alloy using Taguchi method. *Engineering Science and Technology, an International Journal*, 18(4), 524–535.

[15] Almacinha, J., Lopes, A., Rosa, P., & Marafona, J. (2018). How hydrogen dielectric strength forces the work voltage in the electric discharge machining. *Micromachines*, 9(5), 240.

[16] Tseng, K.-H., Chiu, J.-L., Lee, H.-L., Liao, C.-Y., Lin, H.-S., & Kao, Y.-S. (2015). Preparation of Ag/Cu/Ti nanofluids by spark discharge system and its control parameters study. Advances in Materials Science and Engineering, 2015, 1–10.

[17] Al-Shatty, W., Lord, A. M., Alexander, S., & Barron, A. R. (2017). Tunable surface properties of aluminum oxide nanoparticles from highly hydrophobic to highly hydrophilic. *ACS Omega*, 2(6), 2507–2514.

[18] Rades, S., Hodoroaba, V.-D., Salge, T., Wirth, T., Lobera, M. P., Labrador, R. H., … Unger, W. E. S. (2014). High-resolution imaging with SEM/T-SEM, EDX and SAM as a combined methodical approach for morphological and elemental analyses of single engineered nanoparticles. *RSC Advances*, 4(91), 49577–49587.

[19] S. K. Das, S.U.S, Choi, W. Yu and T. Pradeep, *Nanofluids: Science and Technology*, Wiley Interscience: pp. 1–397, 2016.

[20] R. Sarathi, T.K. Sindhu and S.R. Chakravarthy, "Generation of nano aluminium powder through wire explosion process and its characterization," *Materials Characterization*, vol. 58 (2), pp. 148–155, May 2014.

[21] Teng, T.-P., Cheng, C.-M., & Pai, F.-Y. (2011). Preparation and characterization of carbon nanofluid by a plasma arc nanoparticles synthesis system. *Nanoscale Research Letters*, 6(1), 293.

[22] Bilal, A., Jahan, M., Talamona, D., & Perveen, A. (2018). Electro-discharge machining of ceramics: A review. *Micromachines*, 10(1), 10.

[23] Shu Xiao, Kolb, J. F., Malik, M. A., Xinpei Lu, Laroussi, M., Joshi, R. P., … Schoenbach, K. H. (2006). Electrical breakdown and dielectric recovery of propylene carbonate. *IEEE Transactions on Plasma Science*, 34(5), 1653–1661.

[24] J. Hemalatha, T. Prabhakaran, and R.P. Nalini, "A comparative study on particle-fluid interactions in micro and nanofluids of aluminium oxide," *Microfluid Nanofluid*, vol. 10, pp. 263–270, Feb. 2015.

[25] H. M. Lee and Y.J. Kim, "Preparation of size-controlled fine Al particles for application to rear electrode of Si solar cells," *Solar Energy Materials and Solar Cells*, vol. 95, pp. 3352–3358, August 2015.

[26] K.-H. Tseng, H.-L. Lee, W.-P. Feng, C.-Y. Liao, and Y.-S. Kao. "Preparation of alumina nanoparticles by electrical discharge machining," *2014 IEEE 9th Conference on Industrial Electronics and Applications (ICIEA)*, pp. 1787–1790, June 2014.

7 Development
of Electrical
Discharge Machining
Servomechanism System
Towards Biomedical
Application

Nor Liyana Safura Hashim, Ahmad Majdi Abdul-Rani, Iqtidar Ahmed Gul, Azli Yahya, Nor Hisham Khamis, Nazriah Mahmud, and Kartiko Nugroho

7.1 INTRODUCTION ELECTRICAL DISCHARGE MACHINING (EDM)

The manufacturing process of orthopaedic implant involves computer numerical controller (CNC) multi-axis machine tools that are able to produce high-quality complex components for materials such as plastic or titanium. During manufacturing of the medical devices, internal stress might be introduced and may cause the characteristics of the material to be distorted [1]. These stresses are a risk to the implant and may lead to an implant failure during implantation which can cause harm to the patient [2].

Therefore, an electro-discharge machining (EDM) has been used in many applications as well as in biomedical field as its ability to machine with high-level accuracy and better surface finish rather than using conventional machining such as in Strasky et al. [3]. Furthermore, EDM machining process does not induce any heat into the workpiece and this reduces stress defects in the manufactured components of biomedical devices. This book chapter will elaborate more on EDM system and the application of EDM in biomedical application.

Generally, conventional machining methods such as milling, grinding, and drilling processes are chosen since the machined materials are relatively softer than the tool materials. However, according to Sen et al. [4], an advancement of technology in this global world requires the use of harder and brittle materials. Since it is necessary that the machining processes improved in their accuracy and its surface finish, several factors such as the surface integrity of materials including its mechanical, physical,

    DOI: 10.1201/9781003456018-7

and metallurgical properties must be taken into considerations in the machining process to reduce defects. Thus, conventional machining is no longer suitable to be used, as they do not provide good performance in machining harder and brittle materials. Furthermore, frequent tool re-sharpening, excessive drill breakage, poor ability of hard alloys to withstand machining, and formation of entry or exit burrs with mechanical drills make other conventional drilling process almost impractical in micro-holes production [5–7].

An EDM is one of the most important machining methods and widely used among the other non-traditional machining methods. EDM or spark erosion is known as a non-traditional machining process to remove an extremely hard and brittle material which cannot be machined using conventional process [4]. As EDM does involve a non-contact process, it could reduce vibration, mechanical stress, and force towards the machining, thus producing higher quality of machined material than conventional machining such as drilling as mechanical drilling process leaves mechanical distortion in the hole, especially at the entrance and exit.

In biomedical devices manufacturing process, the surface should be void of pores, cracks and also must not contain any toxic substances which can harm the human body. Any undesired machining could affect the characteristic of the implant material, giving risk of inflammatory reactions to the patient. It has been known that EDM can create complex shape with high accuracy for hard material and gives a good result in surface finish if compared to conventional methods. Since metallic biomaterials such as magnesium, alloy, titanium, stainless steel, cobalt chrome, etc., are used widely in implant manufacturing due to its characteristic and biocompatibility [8] which is impossible to be machined using conventional machining thus, this medical field is actually rely heavily on EDM machining for the manufacturing process. In addition, the research by Klocke et al. [9] has been conducted by including some modification on EDM system so that it can be used to manufacture medical device with better performance or surface finish.

7.2 EDM AND WORKING PRINCIPLE

An EDM process is based on the spark and thermoelectric energy that is created between a workpiece and an electrode immersed in a dielectric fluid [10]. It is one of the earliest non-traditional processes that was discovered by Lazarenko and Lazarenko in 1943 [7]; in the process of trying to remove a stuck drill bit from a hole by using pulsed electrical discharge. Basically, there are three types of EDM which are wire EDM, die-sinking, and small-hole EDM. This chapter will discuss on die-sinking EDM.

EDM differs from the other machining operations as it does not make any direct contact with the workpiece to remove metal material. The desired shape of workpiece is obtained using electrical discharges (sparks). In this process, electrical energy through sparking frequency is used to remove the materials. During machining, the tool (known as electrode) and the workpiece must be electrically conductive and the gaps between them are filled with a dielectric fluid.

Figure 7.1 shows a block diagram of structure for a die-sinking EDM. For easier understanding, EDM machine can be divided into four parts: power supply or power generator; flushing system; workpiece table, and the controller unit, and servo system.

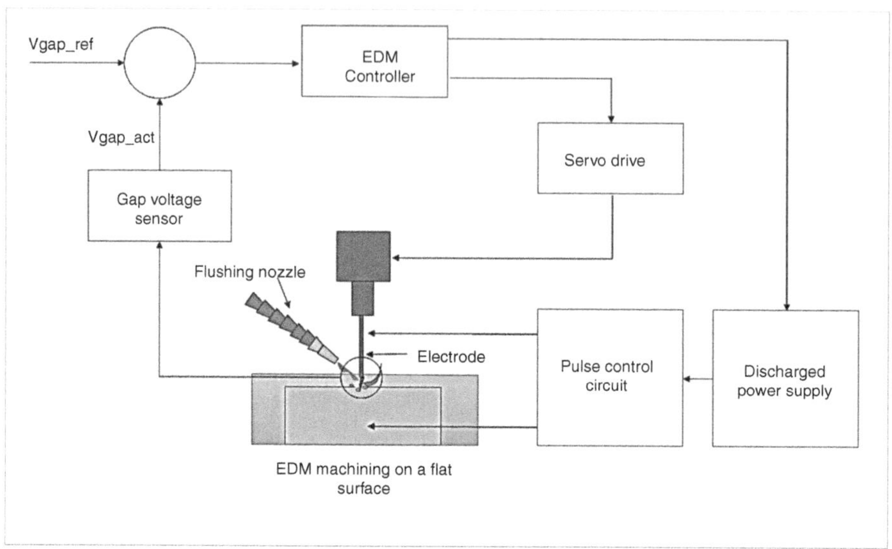

FIGURE 7.1   Basic block diagram of die-sinking EDM.

Each of these parts has their own functions. The focus will be on the EDM servo system, which will be elaborated more on the next section.

Power supply generator produces an electrical spark discharge between the electrode and the workpiece [11]. The generator will control and generate an appropriate machining spark in order to complete the process. As EDM process does not involve physical contact between the electrode and workpiece, it is important that the controller unit and servo system execute mechanical spark adjustment, provide an optimum gap for the efficient machining and prevent electrode from touching the workpiece. If the electrode came into contact with the workpiece, it would create a short-circuit condition in which no machining process occurs. Thus, EDM provides a servo system to control the optimum gap between the electrode and workpiece automatically. Basically, EDM system is categorized into two subsystems which are the servo system and the EDM process. The servo system consists of a multi-loop controller of inner current, speed, and position loops and an outer average voltage loop to ensure an accurate position control of the tool-electrode related to the workpiece. The servo system will determine the error between V_{Gap_ref} and V_{Gap_act} signals and generates the control signal for the servo to position the electrode in z-direction towards the workpiece [14]. The control unit and servo system part are discussed further in the next section. The flushing system function is to remove debris or machined materials from the machining process. EDM is non-sophisticated process, thus this flushing system is important so that the debris or the machined materials do not affect the machining process and machining parameters. Improper flushing could cause an erratic cutting. As the eroded particles accumulate inside the cavity of the machined materials, it could increase the machining time. It also will lead to arcing that could damage of the workpiece. It can be said that the deeper the cavity, greater the difficulty in the flushing system.

Working principle of EDM is not really easy as there are many parameters involved. In EDM, dielectric fluid acts as an insulator until the potential difference is sufficiently high. It allows sufficient current to develop. It also acts as a cooling medium and as flushing medium to remove the debris in the gap. The dielectric medium is usually kerosene or deionized water. For die-sinking, hydrocarbon oil is usually used. The workpiece and tool are connected to a power source which the positive and negative terminal are applied depending upon the desired cutting conditions. Generally, the tool is connected to the positive terminal of the generator, while the workpiece is connected to the negative terminal [12]. During on time of the power supply, an electrical voltage is set up between the workpiece and tool. As dielectric acts as an insulator, there are no current flows, initially. However, when the gap is decreased to a given distance which is very small, the current will flow and the insulating properties of the dielectric fluid will break down. Plasma channel will start to form which the plasma zone could reach up to 8000–12,000°C. The heat causes the fluid to ionize. The spark then occurs between the electrode and workpiece, and can be quite intense at a certain point on the workpiece. Temperature at this spark point on the workpiece will increase. This will cause small quantity of metal to melt and evaporate. Figure 7.2 illustrates the electrode and workpiece in dielectric fluid, an electrical spark between electrode and workpiece, and current profile in sparking gap.

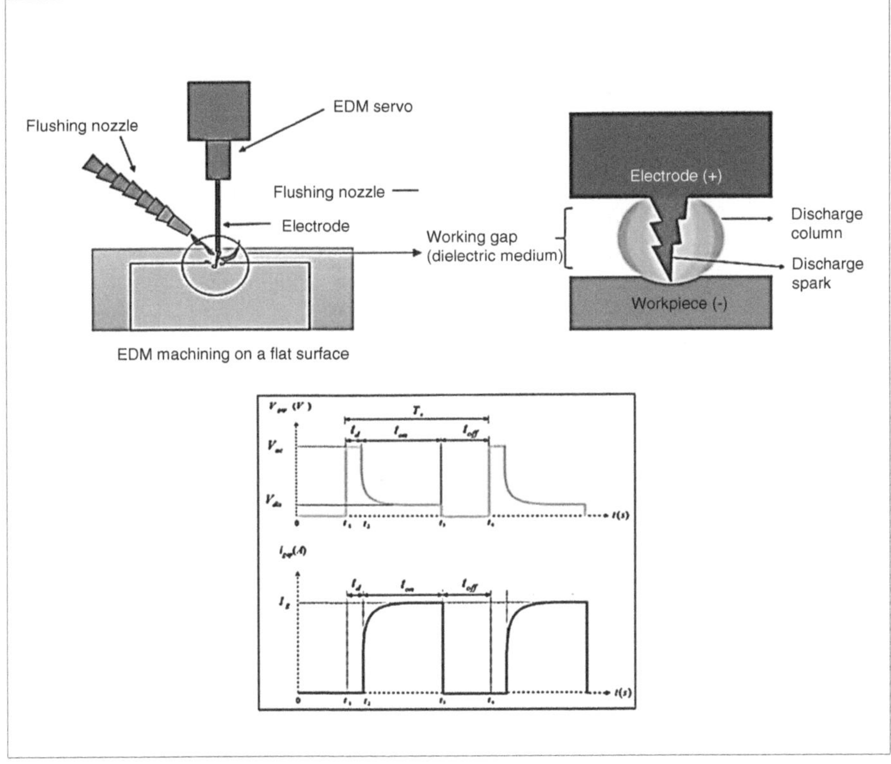

FIGURE 7.2   EDM process.

Whereas during off time, the dielectric oil will cool the vapourized material while the pressurized oil removes the eroded and unwanted machined materials.

From the process, it can be seen that each of the parts play an important role to complete the machining. The dielectric fluid used in EDM provides important functions during EDM process as it acts as a medium for spacing between the electrode and workpiece, as a cooling medium for the heated material to form EDM chip, and as a flushing fluid to remove the eroded particle from the sparking area through flushing system.

7.3 EDM SERVO SYSTEM

It is well-known that EDM is a non-contact process. Therefore, this servo system part of EDM plays an important role to predetermine gap spacing and execute the mechanical spark adjustment in order to achieve an optimum gap between the electrode and the workpiece for proper machining, thus preventing both of them contacting with each other. This mechanism is known as servo-controlled feed mechanism [4] which consists of granite base, three-axis linear platform (X, Y, and Z), and some of them has A-axis rotary table to rotate workpiece at any angle, rotary spindle, and grinding device [13]. The traditional servo mechanism of EDM regulated the motion of the electrode with a brushless DC motor. The simplest control system uses a Z-axis servo drive to maintain a suitable intermediate voltage across the gap during the pulse on period, ensures that discharges are occurring in the correct way [4]. The basic mechanical part of EDM servo system is shown in Figure 7.3 which consists of two

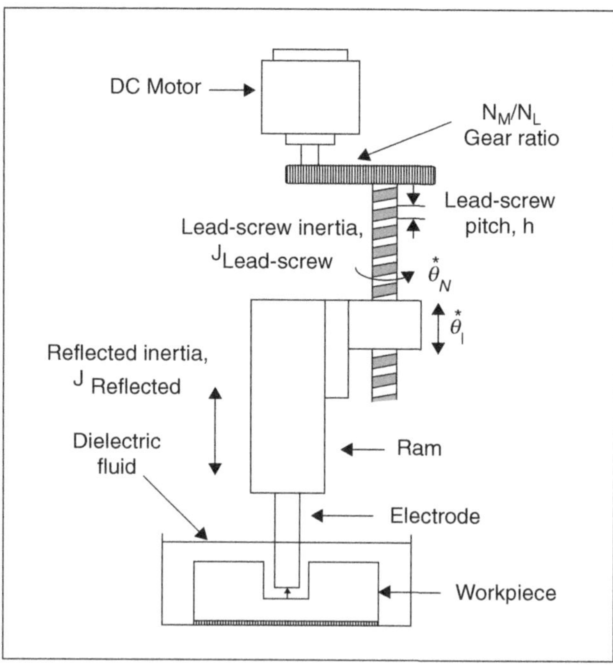

FIGURE 7.3 Servo motor and lead screw load containing the tool electrode.

major subsystems; DC servomotor with controller and a lead-screw containing the tool-electrode.

7.3.1 Tool Feed Drive

In positioning the electrode, lead-screw positioning mechanism are conventionally used in EDM [14], because most of the motion controllers are capable of performing lead-screw compensation. The quality of the lead screws would determine the overall accuracy, while the nut could help to eliminate backlash if it is properly executed. The lead screw would give adequately performance in electrode positioning system and it is able to serve as the linear actuating mechanism in majority of positioning system [15]. However, the positioning response of the lead-screw mechanism is quite slow to maintain discharge distance for the machining due to the mass of stacked tables and rotary inertia of the lead screws [16, 17].

During the operation of EDM, the gap between the tool-electrode and workpiece will change continuously, due to the continuously workpiece material removal. Therefore, high speed and high precision and re-positioning of the electrode are required in order to maintain the ideal gap to get an ideal electrical discharge condition. In addition, the debris around the electrode also has to be removed immediately to avoid the abnormal electrical discharge and several research has been conducted to study and improve the debris removing process [18–21]. Instead of using lead screw, research by Hsue and Chung [22] used linear motor to release debris efficiently.

Development of linear motors equipped direct drive EDM and its control strategy for high-speed machining has been done by Liao [23] and Hsue and Chung [24]. In high dynamic applications, linear motor drives also used in precision machining [25]. The mechanism does not require transmission elements to convert rotational movement to translational movements. It is found by Yan and Cheng [26] that this mechanism has less friction, no backlash, less mechanical limitations, acceleration and velocity, higher reliability, and longer lifetime. In addition, due to its simple mechanical arrangement and relatively low cost of linear drive technology, it is widely used as a basis for developing a table motion system for micro-EDM [27].

7.3.2 Servo Control System

Servo-drive control system is an important part in EDM as it functions to maintain the spark-gap between the tool and workpiece at the desired distance. Therefore, several control strategies have been applied in this system in order to ensure a stable and effective machining. In general, all EDM machines use an automatic control in its servomechanism system in which the discharge gap is controlled automatically. During the machining process, the electrode will penetrate into the workpiece and some parameters other than spark gap will change. When this happens, it is necessary to make an adjustment DC to generator setting in order to restore the stable conditions. This process needed to be monitored and adjusted by skilled operators. However, since the machining process involving stochastic process with more parameters that need to be controlled and high-frequency pulses, it will make this operation is extremely difficult [4]. Therefore, an adaptive control strategy is necessary to be implemented in EDM machining which will be able to detect and react to EDM status changes by continuously adjusting system response based on the feedback information [28].

7.3.2.1 ADAPTIVE CONTROL SYSTEM (ACS)

In 1970, an adaptive control system (ACS) was introduced [32]. This system is used to detect an error signal and send the correcting signal to the servo-drive mechanism. The error signal is measured by comparing the ideal output pattern as reference with the actual output. This system improves the machining productivity by almost 50% and avoiding arcing, thus reducing the workpiece damage. The main advantage of using an adaptive controller is the ability to modify its behaviour in response to timely varied gap state in EDM process and to the disturbance. However, in this technique, the process model and the controller parameter need to be determined. Therefore, this system was merged into EDM application providing a self-tuning regulator. It was design to control the EDM operation so that the gap states will follow the specified gap state based on the real-time process [29]. The simulation of ACS in EDM also has been studied by Yang et al. [30]. Recently, Melnik et al. [31] has developed an ACS based on vibroacoustic emission that is more informative to give adequate data about conditions in the working zone and more convenient to be implemented in EDM.

7.3.2.2 Adaptive Control Optimization (ACO)

In 1979, an adaptive control optimization (ACO) technique was introduced which enables the detection of machining trends that lead to unnecessary conditions and take appropriate actions before the conditions really occurred. This system is divided into two categories, offline optimization and online optimization. In offline optimization, optimal selection of parameters such as pulse current, pulse duration, or discharge current need to be set before the machine starts to operate, while in online optimization, several parameters are left for in-process computer optimization and control in order to achieve optimal performance [4].

This system also has been implemented in EDM by Kruth et al. [32] in 1983 using mini computers, EDM-process-analyser sensors and control devices and its interfaces will automatically searches for machine settings coinciding with optimal working conditions. However, EDM process depends on multiple independent parameters that influence each other, making the machining process a typical random multiple parameters and time-variant nonlinear system [33]. Hence, due to poor gap control of the ACO system and the difficulty of online adjustment because of the stochastic, nonlinear, and dynamic process that occurred during EDM machining, fuzzy knowledge system was applied in EDM system in 1995 by Marco [34].

7.3.2.3 Fuzzy System

A fuzzy knowledge system has been used widely in EDM servo-system application as well as in micro-machining because its capability of handling a highly nonlinear process with only qualitative knowledge available and it is well suited in the EDM environment in order to control the gap between the electrode and workpiece. More researches have been made in this control to aid the operators, thus improving the machining process as it has faster response, more robust and higher stability technique [35–39]. During conversion of the state from a non-machining state to a machining state, it is necessary to make sure that the tool-electrode is in a right location. The conversion control of the different machining states is also needed in order to achieve higher efficiency, in which the tool-electrode can be quickly elevated, and accurate and rapid orientation can be realized. Zhang et al. [36] has developed a structure of an adaptive fuzzy control system for EDM combined with ultrasonic vibration. Micro-processor I would receive some controlled parameters of the servomechanism such as feed, stop, and elevation as the position sensor inspects the actual position of the electrode and rapidly controls the orientation of the electrode. The fuzzy control technology is applied to realize the control of the frequency and the step of the servomechanism according to the collected information such as position error and tool movement speed. The step motor used will drive the tool-electrode at decreasing speed as the tool-electrode move closer to the correct discharge gap and vice versa. For the other condition, the step motor will move with a full step and a changed speed.

Although fuzzy logic is able to deal with nonlinear and time-varying nature in EDM process, the discrimination of pulses from RC type power source is still an ill-defined problem relying on heuristic, as it is important to discriminate between different levels of pulses for proper operation in micro EDM machining. Therefore, a tuneable fuzzy logic-based servo controller for monitoring and control the micro-EDM process was developed by Byiringiro et al. [40] in order to provide stable machining which improve the performance. The system has been developed by classifying the discharge pulses through measurement and analysis of voltage and gap current pulse characteristics.

Fuzzy approach also has been implemented by Shabgard et al. [41]. It was developed for better and user friendly to predict MRR, TWR, and surface roughness in the EDM and ultrasonic-assisted EDM process. They found that the proposed model provides more precise and easy selection of EDM input parameters which lead to better machining conditions.

7.3.2.4 P, PI, PD, PID Controller

In modern mechanical systems such in machine tools, a robust, high speed and high accuracy positioning of motion controller is necessary. Speed of response for the system which determines how quickly a system responds to a change in input is also important, in which the performance of the system can be evaluated from the system step response. However, the linear range of the feedback element is generally limited and the saturation feedback element would disturb the control performance during the control process. If the proportional (P) controller is used to control the feedback system, the saturated feedback signals would increase the rise time. The gain value parameter needs to be increased whenever the travelling speed is large. It will lead to substantially unstable system. In order to reduce the instability of the system, Integral (I) controller then can be connected in parallel to the P controller to reduce rise time and eliminating steady-state error. The robust variable structure system using PI/P controller has been developed which can be applied in EDM to achieve high precise positioning system [42].

In motion control, there are two major sources of uncertainties which are friction and inertia [43]. Since the EDM operation needs to deal with random and uncertainty conditions during the machining process, the regulation of variance and stability of the stochastic process in real-time issues will be discussed. It leads to the use of proportional-integral, PI controller in EDM application [44, 45].

In multi-axis system, it is known that each of the axes has its own system dynamics. Therefore, PI controller also has been used in designing control system that involving four-axis position synchronous control [46]. PI velocity servo also used in traditional servo systems as an alternative approach which regards the bounded nonlinear friction term as disturbance. However, an I-action in the system may cause a limited cycle around a target position in point-to-point control and magnifying the tracking error when motion direction is reversed. Therefore, the introduction to proportional-derivative (PD) controller has been made and it was used in Lee and Tomizuka [43] to utilize the linear feedback control theory in order to construct an asymptotically stable position feedback loop.

Proportional-Integral-Derivative (PID) controller was then introduced and has been used in feedback control in most of industry and manufacturing application [47]. It utilizes a predefined mathematical model to dynamically adjust the servo movement according to the feedback sensor and this controller is commonly used in EDM process control [28]. The values of parameters in this controller must be tuned according to the characteristic of the process in order to yield satisfactory results [48], optimally the system performance and improving efficiency in micro-EDM process [49]. This controller also could have been cascaded with differential controller as differential-PID (DPID) that was implemented by Chung et al. [50] as controlling strategy in the beginning and middle stage in die-sinking EDM machining and it increasing the machining efficiencies up to 30%.

PID control with its term's functionality could improve both the transient and steady-state response, thus making it simpler and an efficient alternative to many control problems. Table 3.1 summarizes the effects of increasing each of the PID controller parameters, K_p, K_I, and K_D. However, the processes involved are in general complex and time-variant, with delays and nonlinearity and often with poor dynamic. Thus, due to its simple structure and robustness, it is quite difficult to optimally tune the gains of this controller by conventional approaches of PID controllers [51]. Therefore, over the years, several researches have proposed many optimizing methods implemented in PID controller specifically in EDM application such as

TABLE 7.1

The effects of increasing each of controller parameters K_p, K_I, and K_D [56]

Response	Rise time	Overshoot	Settling time	S-S error
K_p	Decrease	Increase	NT	Decrease
K_I	Decrease	Increase	Increase	Eliminate
K_D	NT	Decrease	Decrease	NT
*** NT: No definite trend, minor change**				

genetic algorithms [52], particle swarms optimization [53, 54], and also differential evolutions [55].

7.4 EDM IN BIOMEDICAL APPLICATION

As EDM offered better surface finishing and quality, it has been widely used in various applications such as in aerospace, automotive component, and also in biomedical. For example, in biomedical, EDM has been proven to improve surface properties of implants by mean of healing time and bone formation. It is reported that the superimposed topography surface produced by EDM could provide a more suitable surface and potential for osteoblastic cell attachment. It also been reported that cell is highly adopted the specimen treated by EDM after 24 h of cell culture time [57].

7.4.1 SURFACE TEXTURING IN HIP IMPLANT

In hip implant area, several researches have been conducted on the effects of hip implant to patients [58, 59] and has been reviewed [60]. It was observed that the MoM hips articulation still suffers from wear and friction due to the moving metal surface, thus shortening the survival of the joint. Therefore, surface texturing (which also can be define as dimple, oil pockets, or holes) was proposed for lubrication purpose, which eventually prolong the lifespan of the hip implant.

Surface texturing was found to improve tribology properties of journal bearings by reducing friction in two ways, providing lift as a micro-hydrodynamic bearing and acting as a reservoir of lubricant [61–65]. It has been shown experimentally that surface texturing could reduce wear and friction between the contact surface between acetabular and head component in hip implant [66–69]. Figure 7.4 illustrates how the surface texturing was proposed to be machined on hip implant devices. The beneficial of the dimple formation in hip implant application also has been studied by a numerical and simulation [70].

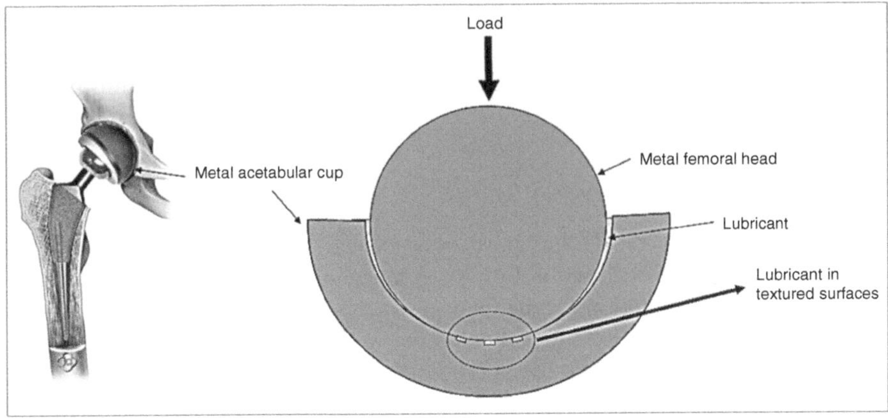

FIGURE 7.4 Dimple on the hip implant.

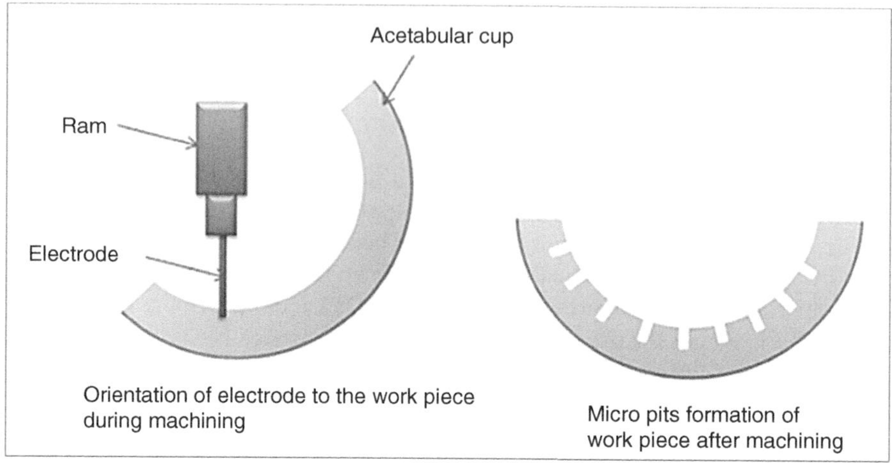

FIGURE 7.5   Machining method of surface texturing on acetabular cup of hip implant.

7.4.2 Manufacturing the Textured Surface

The dimple formation involves a micro-machining process. For this medical purpose, the machining process need to be precise, accurate, and could produce good surface finish with less deterioration on the machined materials. Thus, conventional machining such as milling, grinding, and drilling process are no longer suitable. As EDM is a non-contact process between electrode and workpiece, mechanical stresses and chatters vibration during machining can be eliminated and deterioration of the workpiece structure can be reduced.

However, hip implant devices (especially the acetabular cup) have a spherical surface in which a specially designed and control-method for workpiece positioning system is needed in order to machine the pits perpendicular to the spherical surface such as shown in Figure 7.5. Thus, some modification on existing EDM workpiece positioning system needs to be done, as the conventional workpiece positioning system has a large axis number and not suitable to handle spherical surface. Therefore, Hashim et al. [71, 72] proposed a new multiple axis workpiece positioning system which is suitable to machining micro-pits on the hip implants using EDM.

7.4.3 Workpiece Positioning System

As mentioned earlier, researches have been conducted to develop the workpiece positioning system to machine a dimple on acetabular cup of hip implant. In this design, a swing and rotation mechanism of the system is chosen. This mechanical system is provided with an adjustable clamper to hold the workpiece (hip implant), a mechanism to make sure that the position of the workpiece is accurate so that the pits can be machined perpendicularly to the curvy workpiece surface, a mechanism to make sure that the workpiece is positioned at the centre of the rotation axis, and minimizing the manufacturing cost in terms of the shape, mass, and material used. Figure 7.6 shows the overall workpiece positioning system that was developed while Figure 7.7 shows: (a) implementation of the system to the EDM machine

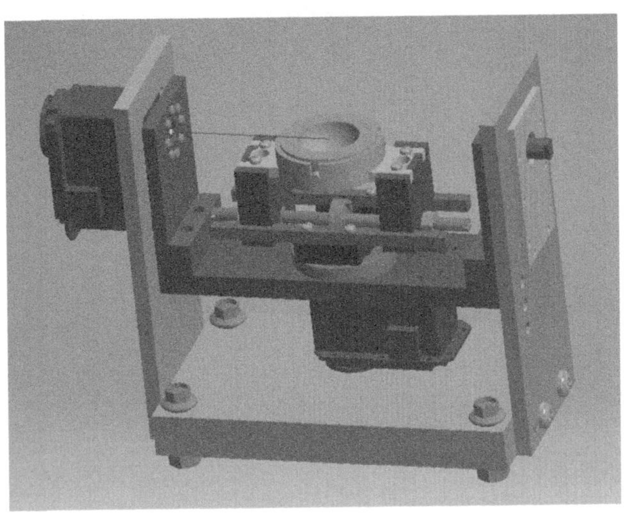

FIGURE 7.6   Overall Workpiece positioning system.

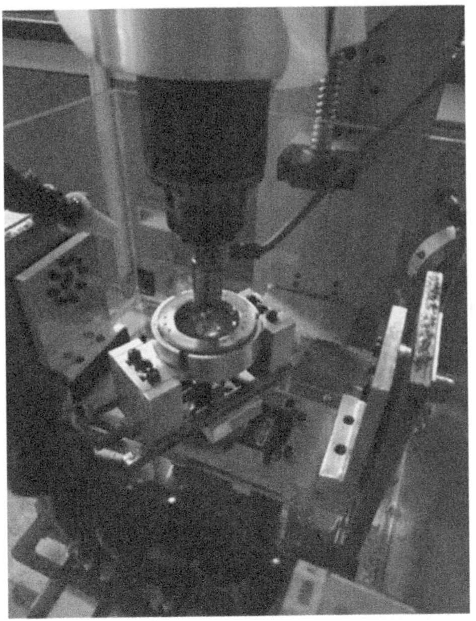

FIGURE 7.7   (a) Machining dimple on acetabular cup of hip implant using developed workpiece positioning system. (b) Acetabular cup with textured surface.

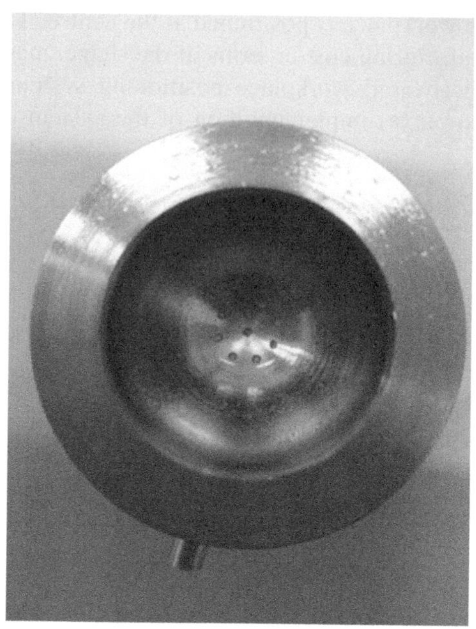

FIGURE 7.7 (Continued)

to machine the dimples on the acetabular cup and (b) the product. The system was provided with its own graphical user interface to set the distance between each dimples formed [73].

7.5 CONCLUSIONS

It has been known that EDM can create complex shape with high accuracy for hard material and gives a good surface finish compared to conventional methods. Metallic biomaterials such as magnesium, alloy, titanium, stainless steel, and cobalt chrome are widely used in implant manufacturing due to their characteristics and biocompatibility. However, they are impossible to be machined using conventional machining. Thus, this medical field actually is relying heavily on EDM machining for the manufacturing process.

In order to maintain proper machining characteristic and performance, it is necessary to make sure that the optimum discharge gap between electrode and workpiece is achieved. This can be done by choosing the right servomechanism and control strategies that is suitable with the application and desired product. For the EDM control strategies, it is necessary to choose the right type of controller for controlling the process while feed drive systems and its mechanical properties are important to provide smooth movements and improved machining time. As EDM is non-sophisticated and complicated process, there are interests to conduct further study and research in order to get a better knowledge about this machining.

ACKNOWLEDGMENTS

Authors would like to acknowledge Research Management Center (RMC) in Universiti Teknologi Malaysia (UTM) for financial support (Vot R.J130000.7651.4C374). Authors also would like to gratitude a special work by technical staff in UTM for their technical help and cooperation.

REFERENCES

[1] Sridhar, G., Volume of material removal on distortion in machining thin wall thin floor components. *Int. J. Mech. Eng. Appl.* 2015, 3, 86.

[2] Prasad, K., Bazaka, O., Chua, M., Rochford, M., et al., Metallic biomaterials: current challenges and opportunities. *Materials (Basel).* 2017, 10.

[3] Strasky, J., Havlikova, J., Bacakova, L., Harcuba, P., et al., Characterization of electrical discharge machining, subsequent etching and shot-peening as a surface treatment for orthopedic implants. *Appl. Surf. Sci.* vol. 281, 2013, pp. 73–78. doi:10.1016/j.apsusc.2013.02.053.

[4] Sen, B., Kiyawat, N., Singh, P.K., Mitra, S., et al., in:, *Power Electron. Drive Syst. 2003. PEDS 2003. Fifth Int. Conf.*, vol. 2, 2003, pp. 998–1003.

[5] Miranda-giraldo, M., Serje-martínez, D., Pacheco-bolívar, J., Bris-cabrera, J., *Burr formation and control for polymers micro-milling: A case study with vortex tube cooling • Formación de rebabas y su control para el micro-fresado de polímeros: Un caso de estudio con refrigeración por tubo vortex* 2017, 84, 150–159.

[6] Costa, E.S., Bacci, M., Machado, A.R., Burr produced on the drilling process as a function of tool wear and lubricant-coolant conditions. *J. Brazilian Soc. Mech. Sci. Eng.* 2009, XXXI, 57–63.

[7] Hebbar, R.R., Ramabadhran, R., Chandrasekar, S., *Hybrid Servomechanism for Micro-Electrical Discharge Machining*, 2002.

[8] Hendra, H., Dadan, R., R.P, D.J., Metals for biomedical applications. *Biomed. Eng. – From Theory to Appl.* 2011, 411–431.

[9] Klocke, F., Schwade, M., Klink, A., Kopp, A., EDM machining capabilities of magnesium (Mg) alloy WE43 for medical applications. *Procedia Eng.* 2011, 19, 190–195.

[10] Pham, D.T., Dimov, S.S., Bigot, S., Ivanov, A., Popov, K., Micro-EDM—recent developments and research issues. *J. Mater. Process. Technol.* 2004, 149, 50–57.

[11] Brick, D., *EDM: Principles of Operation* n.d.

[12] Mahendran, S., Ramasamy, D., Micro-EDM: Overview and recent developments. *Natl. Conf. Mech. Eng. Res. Postgrad. Students (1st NCMER 2010)* 2010, 480–494.

[13] Grabon, W., Koszela, W., Pawlus, P., Ochwat, S., Improving tribological behaviour of piston ring-cylinder liner frictional pair by liner surface texturing. *Tribol. Int.* 2013, 61, 102–108.

[14] Yahya, A., Manning, C.D., Modelling, simulation and controller design for electro discharge machine system. *Electron. Syst. COntorl Div. Res. 2003* 2003.

[15] McCarthy, K., in:, *Motion Control Technol. Conf. Proc., Boston, Mass.,* 1991.

[16] Varanasi, K.K., Nayfeh, S.A., The dynamics of lead-screw drives: low-order modeling and experiments. *J. Dyn. Syst. Meas. Control* 2004, 126, 388.

[17] Zhang, X., Shinshi, T., Endo, H., Shimokohbe, A., et al., in:, *Mechatronics Autom. 2007. ICMA 2007. Int. Conf.,* 2007, pp. 2877–2882.

[18] Liu, Y., Chang, H., Zhang, W., Ma, F., et al., Study on gap flow field simulation in small hole machining of ultrasonic assisted EDM. *IOP Conf. Ser. Mater. Sci. Eng.* 2017, 280.

[19] Wang, J., Han, F., Simulation model of debris and bubble movement in electrode jump of electrical discharge machining. *Int. J. Adv. Manuf. Technol.* 2014, 74, 591–598.

[20] Liu, Y., Chang, H., Zhang, W., Ma, F., et al., A simulation study of debris removal process in ultrasonic vibration assisted electrical discharge machining (EDM) of deep holes. *Micromachines* 2018, 9.

[21] Ho, K.H., Newman, S.T., State of the art electrical discharge machining (EDM). *Int. J. Mach. Tools Manuf.* 2003, 43, 1287–1300.

[22] Hsue, A.W.J., Chung, C.H., Control strategy for high speed electrical discharge machining (die-sinking EDM) equipped with linear motors. *IEEE/ASME Int. Conf. Adv. Intell. Mechatronics, AIM* 2009, 326–331.

[23] Liao, Y.S., Study of debris exclusion effect in linear motor equipped die-sinking EDM process. *Procedia CIRP 6* 2013, 123–128.

[24] Hsue, A.W.-J., Chung, C.-H., in:, *Adv. Intell. Mechatronics, 2009. AIM 2009. IEEE/ASME Int. Conf.*, 2009, pp. 326–331.

[25] Renton, D., Elbestawi, M.A., Motion control for linear motor feed drives in advanced machine tools. *Int. J. Mach. Tools Manuf.* 2001, 41, 479–507.

[26] Yan, M.-T., Cheng, T.-H., High accuracy motion control of linear motor drive wire-EDM machines. *Int. J. Adv. Manuf. Technol.* 2009, 40, 918–928.

[27] Rui, G., Wansheng, Z., Gang, L., in:, *Technol. Innov. Conf. 2006. ITIC 2006. Int.*, 2006, pp. 705–709.

[28] Kao, C.-C., *Monitoring and Control of Micro-Hole Electrical Dishcarge Machining.* The University of Michigan, Ann Arbor, 2007.

[29] Zhou, M., Han, F., Adaptive control for EDM process with a self-tuning regulator. *Int. J. Mach. Tools Manuf.* 2009, 49, 462–469.

[30] Yang, Q. Zhao, Zhou, M., Tian, H. Sen, Zhang, H. Sheng, Xu, D. Hui, Simulation of adaptive control strategy for electrical discharge machining process. *J. Shanghai Jiaotong Univ.* 2015, 20, 408–414.

[31] Melnik, Y., Kozochkin, M., Porvatov, A., Okunkova, A., On adaptive control for electrical discharge machining using vibroacoustic emission. *Technologies* 2018, 6, 96.

[32] Kruth, J.P., Snoeys, R., Brussel, H. V, Adaptive control optimization of the EDM process using minicomputers. *Comput. Ind.* 1979, 1, 65–75.

[33] Zhang, Y., in:, *Mach. Learn. Cybern. 2005. Proc. 2005 Int. Conf.*, Vol. 2, 2005, pp. 726–730.

[34] Boccadoro, M., Dauw, D.F., About the application of fuzzy controllers in high performance die-sinking EDM machines. *Ann. CIRP* 1995, 147–150.

[35] Abdalameer, S., *Controlling of EDM Servo System using Fuzzy Logic Controller Controlling of EDM Servo System Using Fuzzy Logic Controller* 2016, 1–6.

[36] Zhang, J.H., Zhang, H., Su, D.S., Qin, Y., et al., Adaptive fuzzy control system of a servomechanism for electro-discharge machining combined with ultrasonic vibration. *J. Mater. Process. Technol.* 2002, 129, 45–49.

[37] Kao, C.-C., Shih, A.J., Miller, S.F., Fuzzy logic control of microhole electrical discharge machining. *J. Manuf. Sci. Eng.* 2008, 130, 64502–64506.

[38] Kao, C.-C., Shih, A.J., Design and tuning of a fuzzy logic controller for micro-hole electrical discharge machining. *J. Manuf. Process.* 2008, 10, 61–73.

[39] Mahdavinejad, R.A., EDM process optimisation via predicting a controller model. *Arch. Comput. Mater. Sci. Surf. Eng.* 2009, 1, 161–167.

[40] Byiringiro, J.B., Ikua, B.W., Nyakoe, G.N., in:, *AFRICON*, 2009, pp. 1–6.

[41] Shabgard, M.R., Badamchizadeh, M.A., Ranjbary, G., Amini, K., Fuzzy approach to select machining parameters in electrical discharge machining (EDM) and ultrasonic-assisted EDM processes. *J. Manuf. Syst.* 2013, 32, 32–39.

[42] Chang, Y.-F., Chen, B.-S., A robust performance variable structure PI/P control design for high precise positioning control systems. *Int. J. Mach. Tools Manuf.* 1995, 35, 1649–1667.

[43] Lee, H.S., Tomizuka, M., Robust motion controller design for high-accuracy positioning systems. *Ind. Electron. IEEE Trans.* 1996, 43, 48–55.

[44] Chang, Y.-F., in:, *Ind. Electron. Soc. 2007. IECON 2007. 33rd Annu. Conf. IEEE*, 2007, pp. 651–658.

[45] Zhang, X., Shinshi, T., Kajiwara, G., Shimokohbe, A., et al., A 5-DOF controlled maglev local actuator and its application to electrical discharge machining. *Precis. Eng.* 2008, 32, 289–300.

[46] Jeong, S.-K., You, S.-S., Precise position synchronous control of multi-axis servo system. *Mechatronics* 2008, 18, 129–140.

[47] Araki, M., in:, *Control Syst. Robot. Autom., vol. 2, Encyclopedia of Life Support System (EOLSS)*, 2010.

[48] Segovia, J.P., Sbarbaro, D., Ceballos, E., An adaptive pattern based nonlinear PID controller. *ISA Trans.* 2004, 43, 271–281.

[49] Olubiwe, M., Uzoechi, L.O., Uchegbu, V.C., Improved electrical discharge machine (EDM) servomechanism controller for machining micro pits. *Int. J. Eng. Res. Technol.* 2016, 5, 2016.

[50] Chung, C., Chao, S.-Y., Lu, M.F., Modeling and control of die-sinking EDM. *Proc. 9th WSEAS Int. Conf. Robot. Control Manuf. Technol.* 2009, 121–129.

[51] Kumar, V., Rana, K.P.S., Gupta, V., Real-time performance evaluation of a fuzzy PI + fuzzy PD controller for liquid-level process. *Int. J. Intell. Control. Syst.* 2008, 13, 89–96.

[52] Urrea-Quintero, J.-H., Hernández-Riveros, J.-A., Muñoz-Galeano, N., in:, *PID Control Ind. Process*, vol. 2, Intech Open, 2018, p. 64.

[53] Majumder, A., Das, P.K., Majumder, A., Debnath, M., An approach to optimize the EDM process parameters using desirability-based multi-objective PSO. *Prod. Manuf. Res.* 2014, 2, 228–240.

[54] Hashim, N.L.S., Yahya, A., Andromeda, T., Kadir, M.R.A., et al., Simulation of PSO-PI controller of DC motor in micro-EDM system for biomedical application. *J. Procedia Eng.* 2012, 41, 805–811.

[55] Andromeda, T., Yahya, A., Samion, S., Baharom, A., Hashim, N.L., *Differential Evolution for Optimization of PID Gain in Electrical* 2012, 37, 293–301.

[56] Zhong, J., *PID Controller Tuning: A Short Tutorial.* Purdue University, Ann Arbor, 2006.

[57] Prakash, C., Kansal, H.K., Pabla, B.S., Puri, S., Aggarwal, A., Electric discharge machining – A potential choice for surface modification of metallic implants for orthopedic applications: A review. *Proc. Inst. Mech. Eng. Part B J. Eng. Manuf.* 2016, 230, 331–353.

[58] Ingham, E., Fisher, J., Biological reactions to wear debris in total joint replacement. *Proc. Inst. Mech. Eng. H.* 2000, 214, 21–37.

[59] Hernández-Rodríguez, M.A.L., Mercado-Solís, R.D., Pérez-Unzueta, A.J., Martinez-Delgado, D.I., Cantú-Sifuentes, M., Wear of cast metal-metal pairs for total replacement hip prostheses. *Wear* 2005, 259, 958–963.

[60] Merola, M., Affatato, S., Materials for hip prostheses: A review of wear and loading considerations. *Materials (Basel).* 2019, 12.

[61] Etsion, I., Modeling of surface texturing in hydrodynamic lubrication. *Friction* 2013, 1, 195–209.

[62] Gropper, D., Wang, L., Harvey, T.J., Hydrodynamic lubrication of textured surfaces: A review of modeling techniques and key findings. *Tribol. Int.* 2016, 94, 509–529.

[63] Jin, Z.M., Dowson, D., A full numerical analysis of hydrodynamic lubrication in artificial hip joint replacements constructed from hard materials. *Proc. Inst. Mech. Eng., C,* 2016, 213, 355–370.

[64] Han, J., Fang, L., Sun, J., Ge, S., Hydrodynamic lubrication of microdimple textured surface using three-dimensional CFD. *Tribol. Trans.* 2010, 53, 860–870.

[65] Hashim, N.L.S., Harun, M.N., Yahya, A., Suri, M.S., Yusof, A.A.M., Effect of textured curved surface on hydrodynamic pressure. *Proc. Asia Int. Conf. Tribol.,* 2018, 180–181.

[66] Choudhury, D., Walker, R., Shirvani, A., Mootanah, R., The influence of honed surfaces on metal-on-metal hip joints. *Tribol. Online* 2013, 8, 195–202.

[67] Roy, T., Choudhury, D., Ghosh, S., Mamat, A. Bin, Pingguan-Murphy, B., Improved friction and wear performance of micro dimpled ceramic-on-ceramic interface for hip joint arthroplasty. *Ceram. Int.* 2015, 41, 681–690.

[68] Razak, D.M., Syahrullail, S., Sapawe, N., Azli, Y., Nuraliza, N., A new tribological approach on metal cup with optimized pits model using spark discharge machine. *Part. Sci. Technol.* 2016, 34, 209–216.

[69] Choudhury, D., Ay Ching, H., Mamat, A. Bin, Cizek, J., et al., Fabrication and characterization of DLC coated microdimples on hip prosthesis heads. *J. Biomed. Mater. Res. – Part B Appl. Biomater.* 2015, 103, 1002–1012.

[70] Gao, L., Yang, P., Dymond, I., Fisher, J., Jin, Z., Effect of surface texturing on the elastohydrodynamic lubrication analysis of metal-on-metal hip implants. *Tribol. Int.* 2010, 43, 1851–1860.

[71] Hashim, N.L.S., Yahya, A., Abdul Kadir, M.R., in:, *2012 Int. Conf. Biomed. Eng.,* 2012.

[72] Hashim, N.L.S., Yahya, A., Nugroho, K., Mahmud, N., Daud, M.R., *Development of Workpiece Positioning System in Electrical Discharge Machining for Biomedical Application* 2013, 848–851.

[73] Kartiko, N., Azli, Y., Nor Liyana, H.S., Syahrullail, S., Razak Daud, M.D., Development of computer-aided EDM for machining micropits on spherical surface of hip implant. *Appl. Mech. Mater.* 2014, 554, 541–545.

8 Influential Process Parameters Associated with Powder-Mixed Electric Discharge Coating Technique Applied to 316L Steel

Iqtidar Ahmed Gul, Ahmad Majdi Abdul-Rani, Azlan Ahmad, Md Al-Amin, and Habib Ahmad

8.1 INTRODUCTION

316L stainless steel is a popular material for biomedical implant applications due to its excellent corrosion resistance, biocompatibility, and mechanical properties. The alloy contains 10–14% nickel, 17–19% chromium, and 2–3% molybdenum, giving it high corrosion resistance and pitting in biological environments [1]. 316L steel bioimplants are commonly used in orthopaedic, cardiovascular, and dental applications.

One of the challenges associated with 316L steel bioimplants is the potential for corrosion and wear, which can lead to implant failure and adverse patient reactions [2, 3]. Several coating approaches have been explored to increase 316L steel bioimplant surface characteristics. Coatings improve wear, corrosion, biocompatibility, and osseointegration [4]. The proper coating technique and process variables are essential to achieve the necessary features. To coat 316L steel bioimplants, for instance, sol-gel, electrochemical deposition, and plasma spraying have all been tried, but each technique has benefits and drawbacks [5]. Additionally, selecting process variables like coating thickness, deposition temperature, and chemical composition may significantly impact the coating's characteristics.

Statistical analysis may help improve the coating process and find crucial factors influencing coating qualities. This study may assist in finding the best process conditions for achieving the required coating characteristics, minimising coating process variability, and increasing coating material uniformity [6]. Because of its high mechanical qualities and biocompatibility, 316L steel bioimplants are extensively

DOI: 10.1201/9781003456018-8

employed in medical applications. However, corrosion and wear are still significant issues that may lead to implant failure and negative patient responses. Coating techniques have been developed to solve these challenges, and statistical analysis may be a helpful tool for optimising the coating process and finding the essential process factors that determine the coating qualities.

Bioimplants replace, restore, or sustain injured tissue or organs. These devices must be biocompatible, strong, durable, and corrosion-resistant. Coatings increase bioimplant performance, biocompatibility, and usefulness. Bioimplant coating entails covering the implant with a thin substance. Physical vapour deposition (PVD), chemical vapour deposition (CVD), electroplating, and sol-gel coating may apply the coating. Each approach has pros and cons; the coating and implant qualities determine the procedure [7].

PVD coatings are frequently employed in the biomedical sector because of their biocompatibility, corrosion resistance, and wear resistance. These coatings are often applied in a vacuum chamber, allowing for exact control of coating thickness and composition. On the other hand, the expensive cost of PVD equipment and the restricted selection of coating materials might be a disadvantage. CVD coatings, which provide comparable advantages to PVD coatings, have also been employed in the biomedical sector. Contrarily, CVD coatings need high temperatures and pressures, which may limit their suitability for certain implant types. Electroplating is a low-cost method of covering an implant's surface with various metals. Electroplated coatings, on the other hand, are often porous and have poor adhesion to the substrate, which might reduce implant performance. Sol-gel coatings are a more recent coating method that offers good biocompatibility and can include bioactive substances in the coating. Conversely, sol-gel coatings may be fragile and have poor substrate adhesion [8].

Powder-mixed electric discharge coating (PM-EDC) is an emerging technology that deposits a coating on a substrate using electrical discharges in a dielectric liquid medium [9]. This research effort optimised coating process parameters using statistical analysis and PM-EDC. Coating technique and process characteristics affect bioimplant performance. A statistical study of the process parameters for coating 316L Steel bioimplants may assist in determining the best parameters for bioimplants with unique specifications.

In this research study, the data sources were mainly assessed from the journal articles [10,11] for the experimental results concerning the powder-mixed electric charge coating method for 316L steel biomaterial. The influential process factors of the 316L steel coating method have been identified through a statistical tool named Minitab resulting in the enhancement of deposited layer properties such as surface roughness (SR) and micro-hardness.

## 8.2	INFLUENTIAL PROCESS PARAMETERS IN THE PM-EDC PROCESS

The following describes the function of the significant process parameters in the PM-EDC method:

8.2.1 Dielectric Medium

PM-EDC uses a dielectric medium as a process parameter to improve coating productivity and quality. During the coating procedure, the dielectric medium, a nonconductive liquid or gas, fills the gap between the powder mixture and the substrate. Electrical discharge between the powder and the substrate affects coating quality and thickness, which the dielectric medium regulates.

The PM-EDC technique creates an electric spark between the powder combination and the substrate, which then causes the powder to melt and deposit itself locally onto the substrate. The dielectric medium influences coating quality and thickness by stabilising the electrical discharge and regulating the plasma output.

The microstructure and characteristics of the deposited coating may be modified by the dielectric medium, which also influences the substrate's heat transmission and cooling rate. The substrate's cooling rate may be increased, leading to a finer-grained microstructure and higher hardness in the deposited coating when water is used as the dielectric medium. Deionised water, kerosene, ethanol, and mineral oil commonly employ dielectric media in PM-EDC experiments. The substrate and powder material qualities and the required characteristics of the deposited coating determine the dielectric medium to be used. Umair et al. [12] reported the usage of bio-dielectrics for environmentally friendly and sustainable electric discharge machining processes. The research finding discovers that polanga oil and palm styrene extracts are the most influential bio-dielectrics for improving material removal rate (MRR) and SR.

8.2.2 Discharge Current

Discharge current is a critical operational variable in PM-EDC technology. It controls the temperature and energy input into the coating process, determining its final characteristics. Localised melting and powder deposition on the substrate surface come from an electrical spark created by the discharge current in PM-EDC. The properties of the PM-EDC process, such as deposition rate, coating thickness, microstructure, etc., are affected by the discharge current. The deposition rate, coating thickness, and perhaps porosity, roughness, and hardness may all be improved by increasing the discharge current. However, a slower deposition rate and thinner coating may come by using a lower discharge current, which may also provide a denser, smoother, and more lasting coating.

Many aspects, including the substrate and powder combination material quality, the desired coating thickness and properties, and the experimental circumstances, influence the ideal discharge current for PM-EDC. The discharge current may be regulated by altering the voltage and pulse length of the electric discharge, as well as the dielectric medium's electrical and thermal characteristics. Several investigations have been carried out on the effects of discharge current on the PM-EDC procedure and the features of the deposited coatings. The impact of discharge current on hydroxyapatite mixed electro-discharge machining (EDM) and coating deposition on titanium substrate was studied by Prakash and Uddin [13]. A high discharge current of 15 A in a deionised water dielectric medium resulted in a uniformly coated layer with no cracks on the surface.

8.2.3 Pulse-On Time

The pulse-on time is a critical process variable in the PM-EDC technique. The time required for the powder combination and the substrate to undergo an electrical discharge is described. Pulse-on time regulates the amount of energy and heat introduced to the coating process, affecting the coating's properties and quality.

The pulse-on time affects the PM-EDC process parameters, such as the deposition rate, coating thickness, and microstructure. Longer pulse-on periods result in faster deposition and thicker coating, but the resulting layer is more porous, abrasive, and less durable. A shorter pulse-on duration may result in a slower deposition rate and a thinner coating, but it may also provide a more robust, uniform, and long-lasting coating. Several parameters, including the material characteristics of the substrate and powder combination, the desired coating thickness and attributes, and the experimental settings, affect the ideal pulse-on time for PM-EDC. The pulse-on time may be altered by adjusting the voltage, pulse length, and electrical/thermal characteristics of the dielectric media used in the electric discharge.

The impact of pulse-on time on quarry dust mixed EDM and layer deposition on the WC-Co workpiece was reported by Yap et al. [14]. An optimum value of $T_{on} = 341$ µs achieved a hard surface, thickly coated layer, and low surface finish on the substrate.

8.2.4 Pulse-Off Time

The pulse-off time is a crucial process parameter in PM-EDC technology. It measures the intervals between the coating process's electrical discharges. The quality and properties of the deposited coating are affected by the pulse-off time, which controls its cooling and solidification.

Microstructure, porosity, and coating characteristics are all impacted by the pulse-off time in PM-EDC. The coating's microstructure becomes more uniform, dense, and homogenous with reduced porosity and increased hardness as the pulse-off duration increases. The coating microstructure may become more porous and heterogeneous, with decreased hardness and adhesion strength when the pulse-off duration is shorter.

Various parameters influence the ideal pulse-off time for PM-EDC, including the material properties of the substrate and powder combination, the desired coating microstructure and attributes, and the experimental circumstances. The pulse-off time may be modified by altering the voltage and pulse length of the electric discharge.

Multiple investigations have been carried out to learn how the pulse-off time affects the PM-EDC procedure and the characteristics of the deposited coatings. One of the research studies, Tyagi et al. [15] stated that too small a pulse-off time may provide insufficient flushing of debris in the discharge gap during the machining process resulting in a high probability of arching.

8.2.5 VOLTAGE

In the PM-EDC method, voltage is a crucial process parameter. In the context of powder coating, it describes the difference in electrical potential between the powder mixture and the substrate. The voltage regulates the discharge's kinetic energy and the coating's quality.

Voltage has an impact on a variety of PM-EDC process variables, including coating shape, microstructure, and characteristics. A greater voltage causes an increase in energy input and electrical discharge intensity, which speeds up deposition and thickens the coating. A high voltage, on the other hand, might cause the powder particles to arc, melt, and splatter, creating a porous and heterogeneous coating with poor adherence and mechanical strength. On the other side, a lower voltage may lead to a slower deposition rate and a thinner coating, but it will also produce a coating microstructure that is more uniform and denser.

Numerous investigations have been done to determine how voltage affects the PM-EDC process and the characteristics of the deposited coatings. The impact of voltage using nickel tool and layer deposition on the titanium alloy workpiece was reported by Prakash et al. [16]. The research discovers that the parameter voltage significantly affects the recast layer thickness.

8.3 MATERIALS AND METHODS

8.3.1 MATERIALS

A rectangular plate of size 50 mm × 100 mm × 5mm made from biomedical grade steel (316L) was utilised as the workpiece material. A circular bar of 10 mm dia made from pure copper (Cu) was used as the electrode tool. A bio-ceramic powder known as hydroxyapatite (HA) was suspended in the dielectric fluid of EDM to obtain a biocompatible coating on the top surface of the steel. HA powder is preferred in biomedical applications as it possesses bone-like apatite and enhances integration between the implant and surrounding bone tissue. This study assesses the materials and methods from the research articles in Table 8.1.

The elemental composition, material, and mechanical properties of the workpiece, electrode tool, and powder used in the dielectric medium of the electric discharge coating process are provided in Tables 8.2, 8.3, 8.4 and 8.5.

TABLE 8.1

Data sources for assessing the information regarding materials and methods

Data sources	Article	Journal/Publisher
[12]	Surface modification of 316L SS with HAp nano-particles using PM-EDM for enhanced biocompatibility	*Materials Today: Proceedings*/ ELSEVIER
[11]	Surface morphology and micro-hardness behaviour of 316L in HAp-PM-EDM	*Facta Universitatis*/University of Niš

TABLE 8.2
Elemental composition of the workpiece

316L Stainless steel – Workpiece	
Element	**Composition (%)**
Iron (Fe)	63.0–74.0
Chromium (Cr)	16.0–18.0
Nickel (Ni)	10.0–14.0
Molybdenum (Mo)	2.00–3.00
Manganese (Mn)	2.00 max
Silicon (Si)	1.00 max
Carbon (C)	0.03 max
Phosphorus (P)	0.045 max
Sulphur (S)	0.03 max
Nitrogen (N)	0.10 max

TABLE 8.3
Material and mechanical properties of the workpiece

Material/Mechanical properties of 316L stainless steel	Value
Density	8.0 g/cm^3
Elastic modulus	193 GPa
Poisson's ratio	0.3
Thermal conductivity	16.2 W/m·K
Coefficient of thermal expansion	$16.5 \times 10\text{-}6$ /K
Melting point	1399–1420 °C
Yield strength (at 0.2% offset)	170–310 MPa
Ultimate tensile strength	485–620 MPa
Elongation at break	40–60%
Hardness (Rockwell B)	70–95

TABLE 8.4
Material properties of the electrode tool

Material properties of copper (Cu) — Electrode tool	Value
Density	8.96 g/cm^3
Elastic modulus	130–140 GPa
Poisson's ratio	0.34
Thermal conductivity	401 W/mK
Coefficient of thermal expansion	$16.5 \times 10\text{-}6$ /K
Melting point	1085 °C
Tensile strength	220–350 MPa
Compressive strength	220–350 MPa
Elongation at break	30–70%
Hardness, Brinell	35–400 HB

TABLE 8.5
Material properties of the powder used in the dielectric medium

Material properties of hydroxyapatite (HA) – powder	Value
Chemical formula	$Ca_5 (PO4)_3 (OH)$
Molecular weight	502.31 g/mol
Density	3.16 g/cm^3
Melting point	1550 °C
Thermal conductivity	3.15 W/mK
Young's modulus	100–120 GPa
Compressive strength	200–300 MPa
Tensile strength	40–50 MPa
Flexural strength	100–150 MPa
Solubility in water	0.009 g/100 mL (25 °C)

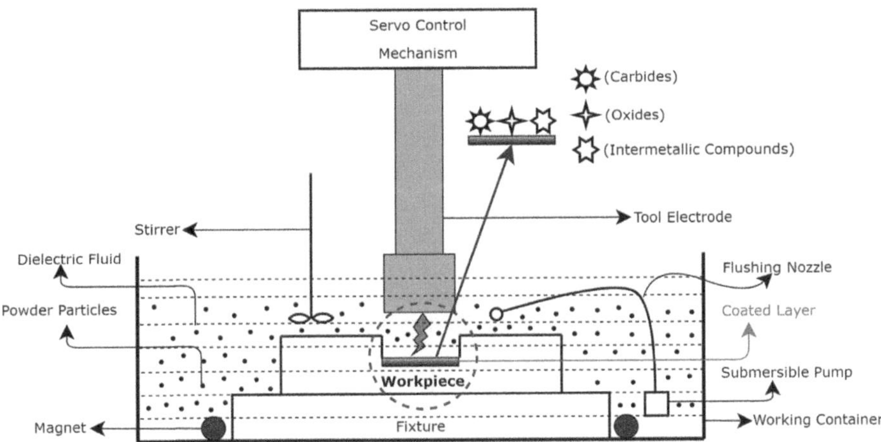

FIGURE 8.1 Power-mixed electric discharge machining and coating process [18] (CC BY 4.0).

8.3.2 Methods

In this study, the PM-EDC method has been considered to evaluate process factors, as this method is still at the early stage of experimental research. The data sources have been extracted from the journal articles tabulated in Table 8.1. PM-EDC is a surface modification technique used for biomedical applications, which involves depositing a coating of a metallic or ceramic powder onto a substrate using electric discharge. This technique offers several advantages, such as improved wear resistance, corrosion resistance, and biocompatibility, making it an attractive option for biomedical implants.

A metallic or ceramic powder is combined with dielectric fluid and then brought into contact with the substrate during the PM-EDC process. As seen in Figure 8.1,

TABLE 8.6
Variable process factors of the PM-EDC process

	Variable process factors				
Sr. No.	Factors	Level	Value		
1	Dielectric medium	2	EDM Oil	EDM Oil + powder	-
2	Discharge current (A)	3	20	24	28
3	Pulse-on time (μs)	3	60	90	120
4	Pulse-off time (μs)	3	60	90	120
5	Voltage (V)	3	40	60	80

an electric spark is created between the powder mixture and the substrate, resulting in localised melting and deposition of the powder onto the substrate surface. The characteristics of the deposited layer may be modified by adjusting process parameters such as dielectric medium, discharge current, pulse-on time, pulse-off time, and voltage. PM-EDC has been used to deposit coatings of numerous materials on biomedical implants, including titanium, titanium alloys, and HA. Al-Amin et al. [6] used the PM-EDC process to coat 316L steel with HA powder. The research claims a thin recast layer with moderate SR as the HA coating considerably increased the bioactivity and biocompatibility of the 316L steel, making it a good option for orthopaedic implants. Singh et al. [17] employed the PM-EDC approach in a TiO_2 nano-powder mixed dielectric medium to evaluate the surface of 316L steel. From the research study, it was found that the addition of nano-powders in the dielectric medium increases the machining stability and material migration.

This study utilised Taguchi L18 orthogonal array mixed-level design ($2^1 \times 3^4$) using a Minitab software statistical tool. The primary purpose is to optimise product or process design by identifying the optimal levels of multiple variables. The L18 Orthogonal Array is an 18-run mixed-level design that allows for the simultaneous study of up to eight factors with different significance levels, including main effects and interactions, with a minimum number of experimental runs. The mixed-level design allows for a combination of discrete and continuous variables and enables the study of nominal and ordinal variables in the same experiment. Referring to the data sources, there are a total of five factors, of which one factor has two levels, whereas rest four factors have three levels and is represented in Table 8.6.

The design summary from the Taguchi design using Minitab software can be tabulated in Table 8.7 in the following manner.

SR and micro-hardness are the crucial properties of the deposited layer on the top surface of the biomaterial, as it provides enhanced bioactivity and biocompatibility. Table 8.7 represents the design summary of 18 experiments with various input factors corresponding to respective outcomes. The experimental data concerning SR and micro-hardness has been extracted from the referred sources.

TABLE 8.7
Design summary with inputs factors (C1– C5) and output responses (C6– C7).

Taguchi Design

Design Summary

Taguchi Array   L18(2^1 3^4)
Factors: 5
Runs: 18

↓	C1	C2	C3	C4	C5	C6	C7
	Dielectric medium	Discharge current (A)	Pulse-on time (µs)	Pulse-off time (µs)	Voltage (V)	Surface Roughness (Ra)	Microhardness (HV)
5	1	24	90	90	80	0.780	538.9
6	1	24	120	120	40	0.923	515.9
7	1	28	60	90	40	0.910	475.2
8	1	28	90	120	60	1.236	374.3
9	1	28	120	60	80	0.846	459.7
10	2	20	60	120	80	0.426	819.4
11	2	20	90	60	40	0.456	557.8
12	2	20	120	90	60	0.983	859.4
13	2	24	60	90	80	0.266	636.2
14	2	24	90	120	40	0.326	663.1
15	2	24	120	60	60	0.733	904.3
16	2	28	60	120	60	0.956	904.6
17	2	28	90	60	80	0.576	779.5
18	2	28	120	90	40	1.296	958.3

8.4   RESULTS AND DISCUSSION

8.4.1   SURFACE ROUGHNESS

SR is crucial in successfully integrating bioimplants with the surrounding tissue. The impact of process factors on the SR of powder-mixed electric discharge-coated samples can be illustrated in Figures 8.2 and Table 8.8.

The smaller SR value is desirable for biomedical applications, and its effectiveness with process factors is shown above. From the results for SR, it has been observed that dielectric medium with only EDM oil, discharge current with 28A, pulse-on time with 120 µs, pulse-off time with 90 µs, and voltage with 60V is recommended. As per the ranking, voltage is first, followed by dielectric medium, discharge current, pulse-on time, and pulse-off time.

8.4.2   MICRO-HARDNESS

Micro-hardness is an important property to consider when developing coatings for bioimplants, as it affects the wear resistance and durability of the implant. The impact of process factors on the micro-hardness of powder-mixed electric discharge-coated samples can be illustrated in Figures 8.4 and Table 8.9.

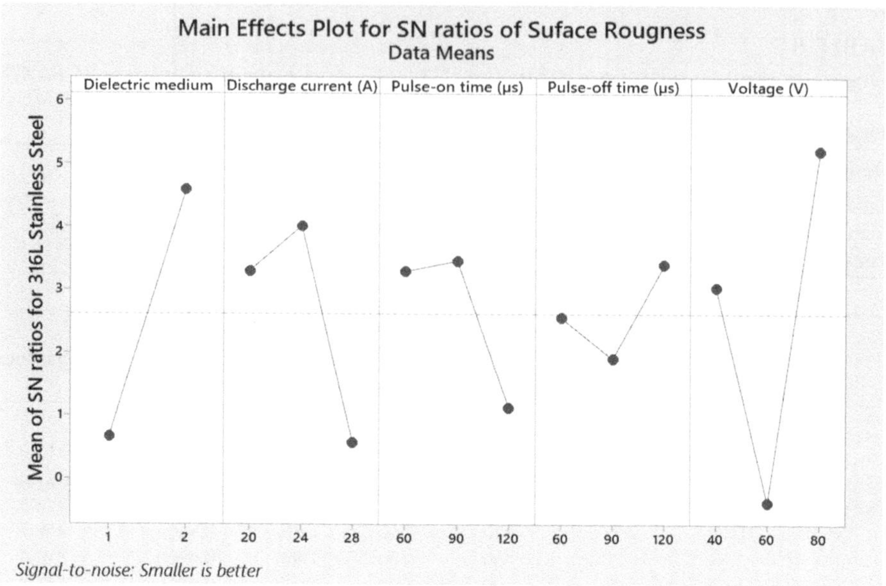

FIGURE 8.2 SN ratios of surface roughness against the five input factors.

TABLE 8.8
Ranking of the influential process factors for surface roughness.

Response Table for Signal to Noise Ratios

Smaller is better

Level	Dielectric medium	Discharge current (A)	Pulse-on time (µs)	Pulse-off time (µs)	Voltage (V)
1	0.6535	3.2916	3.2836	2.5567	3.0281
2	4.5831	4.0029	3.4521	1.9039	-0.3881
3		0.5603	1.1192	3.3943	5.2147
Delta	3.9296	3.4427	2.3329	1.4904	5.6028
Rank	2	3	4	5	1

The larger micro-hardness value is desirable for biomedical applications, and its effectiveness with process factors is shown here. From the results for micro-hardness, it has been observed that dielectric medium with EDM oil and powder, discharge current with 28 A, pulse-on time with 120 µs, pulse-off time with 120 µs, and voltage of 40 V is recommended. As per the ranking, the dielectric medium is first, followed by discharge current, pulse-on time, voltage, and pulse-off time.

8.5 CONCLUSION AND FURTHER STUDY DIRECTIONS

This study aimed to identify the critical process parameters that significantly influence the quality of coatings applied to 316L steel bioimplants using the powder-mixed

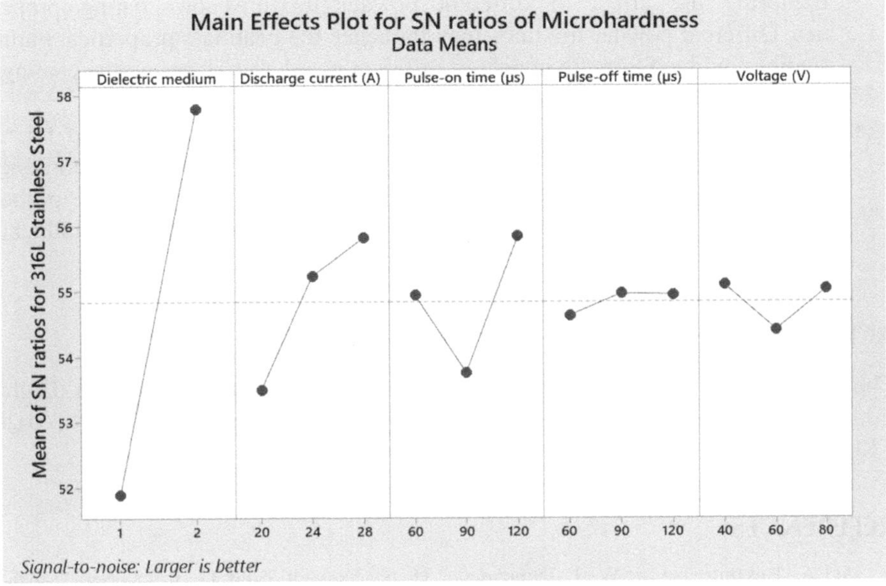

FIGURE 8.4 SN ratios of micro-hardness against the five input factors.

TABLE 8.9
Ranking of the influential process factors for micro-hardness.

Response Table for Signal to Noise Ratios

Larger is better

Level	Dielectric medium	Discharge current (A)	Pulse-on time (µs)	Pulse-off time (µs)	Voltage (V)
1	51.88	53.48	54.93	54.62	55.09
2	57.79	55.22	53.74	54.95	54.40
3		55.81	55.84	54.94	55.02
Delta	5.91	2.33	2.09	0.33	0.69
Rank	1	2	3	5	4

electric discharge coating method. Using the statistical tool Taguchi via Minitab software to analyse data sources collected from journal articles, the study successfully identified the optimal levels of each process parameter, resulting in the deposited layer's desired SR and micro-hardness. The results provide insights into the relationship between process parameters and coating properties, which can be used to enhance the understanding of the coating process and optimise it further. Ultimately, this study contributes to developing better-quality bioimplants, benefiting patients and the medical industry.

Further study directions for this project could include the following:

- Investigating the long-term stability and biocompatibility of the coatings: While this study focused on improving the SR and micro-hardness of coatings, it would be beneficial to investigate their long-term stability and biocompatibility.

- Exploring the effect of different powder mixtures on coating properties: Different powder mixtures may influence the coating's properties. Future studies could explore the impact of different powder mixtures on the coating's SR, micro-hardness, and other properties.
- Optimising other critical properties of the coatings: While SR and micro-hardness are crucial, other properties such as adhesion strength and corrosion resistance are equally important. Future studies could optimise these properties by identifying the essential process parameters that significantly influence them.

ACKNOWLEDGMENTS

The authors express their deep gratitude to the Malaysian Ministry of Higher Education for providing the research work opportunity via a grant (FRGS/1/2020/TK0/UTP/02/39).

REFERENCES

[1] A. Bekmurzayeva, W. J. Duncanson, H. S. Azevedo, and D. Kanayeva, "Surface modification of stainless steel for biomedical applications: Revisiting a century-old material," *Mater. Sci. Eng. C*, vol. 93, no. October 2017, pp. 1073–1089, 2018, doi: 10.1016/j.msec.2018.08.049.

[2] C. H. Chang, J. S. Lin, and W. Eugene Roberts, "Failure rates for stainless steel versus titanium alloy infrazygomatic crest bone screws: A single-center, randomized double-blind clinical trial," *Angle Orthod.*, vol. 89, no. 1, pp. 40–46, 2019, doi: 10.2319/012518-70.1.

[3] M. Sivakumar, K. S. Kumar Dhanadurai, S. Rajeswari, and V. Thulasiraman, "Failures in stainless steel orthopaedic implant devices: A survey," *J. Mater. Sci. Lett.*, vol. 14, no. 5, pp. 351–354, 1995, doi: 10.1007/BF00592147.

[4] X. Yan, W. Cao, and H. Li, "Biomedical alloys and physical surface modifications: A mini-review," *Materials (Basel).*, vol. 15, no. 1, 2022, doi: 10.3390/ma15010066.

[5] M. Al-Amin, A. M. Abdul Rani, A. A. Abdu Aliyu, M. A. Abdul Razak, S. Hastuty, and M. G. Bryant, "Powder mixed-EDM for potential biomedical applications: A critical review," *Mater. Manuf. Process.*, pp. 1789–1811, 2020, doi: 10.1080/10426914.2020.1779939.

[6] M. Al-Amin, A. M. Abdul-Rani, R. Ahmed, and T. V. V. L. N. Rao, "Multiple-objective optimization of hydroxyapatite-added EDM technique for processing of 316L-steel," *Mater. Manuf. Process.*, vol. 36, no. 10, pp. 1134–1145, 2021, doi: 10.1080/10426914.2021.1885715.

[7] M. Al-Amin *et al.*, "Investigation of coatings, corrosion and wear characteristics of machined biomaterials through hydroxyapatite mixed-edm process: A review," *Materials (Basel).*, vol. 14, no. 13, pp. 1–33, 2021, doi: 10.3390/ma14133597.

[8] W. S. W. Harun *et al.*, "A comprehensive review of hydroxyapatite-based coatings adhesion on metallic biomaterials," *Ceram. Int.*, vol. 44, no. 2, pp. 1250–1268, 2018, doi: 10.1016/j.ceramint.2017.10.162.

[9] R. Tyagi *et al.*, "Electrical discharge coating a potential surface engineering technique: a state of the art," *Processes*, vol. 10, no. 10, 2022, doi: 10.3390/pr10101971.

[10] G. Singh, Y. Lamichhane, A. Bhui, S. Sidhu, P. Singh, and P. Mukhiya, "Surface morphology and microhardness behavior of 316L in HAp-PMEDM," vol. 17, pp. 445–454, Dec. 2019, doi: 10.22190/FUME190510040S.

[11] Y. Lamichhane, G. Singh, A. S. Bhui, P. Mukhiya, P. Kumar, and B. Thapa, "Surface modification of 316L SS with HAp nano-particles using PMEDM for enhanced biocompatibility," *Mater. Today Proc.*, vol. 15, pp. 336–343, 2019, doi: 10.1016/j.matpr.2019.05.014.

[12] U. Arif, I. Ali Khan, and F. Hassan, "Green and sustainable electric discharge machining: a review," *Adv. Mater. Process. Technol.*, vol. 00, no. 00, pp. 1–75, 2022, doi: 10.1080/2374068X.2022.2108599.

[13] C. Prakash and M. S. Uddin, "Surface modification of β-phase Ti implant by hydroaxyapatite mixed electric discharge machining to enhance the corrosion resistance and in-vitro bioactivity," *Surf. Coatings Technol.*, vol. 326, pp. 134–145, 2017, doi: 10.1016/j.surfcoat.2017.07.040.

[14] C. Y. Yap, P. J. Liew, and J. Wang, "Surface modification of tungsten carbide cobalt by electrical discharge coating with quarry dust powder: an optimisation study," *Mater. Res. Express*, vol. 7, no. 10, p. 106407, 2020, doi: 10.1088/2053-1591/abc09f.

[15] R. Tyagi, A. K. Das, and A. Mandal, "Electrical discharge coating using WS2 and Cu powder mixture for solid lubrication and enhanced tribological performance," *Tribol. Int.*, vol. 120, pp. 80–92, 2018, doi: 10.1016/j.triboint.2017.12.023.

[16] V. Prakash *et al.*, "Surface alloying of miniature components by micro-electrical discharge process," *Mater. Manuf. Process.*, vol. 33, no. 10, pp. 1051–1061, Jul. 2018, doi: 10.1080/10426914.2017.1364755.

[17] G. Singh, S. S. Sidhu, P. S. Bains, and A. S. Bhui, "Surface evaluation of ED machined 316L stainless steel in TiO2 nano-powder mixed dielectric medium," *Mater. Today Proc.*, vol. 18, pp. 1297–1303, 2019, doi: 10.1016/j.matpr.2019.06.592.

[18] I. A. Gul, A. M. Abdul-Rani, M. Al-Amin, and E. Garba, "Elucidating powder-mixed electric discharge machining process, applicability, trends and futuristic perspectives," *Machines*, vol. 11, no. 3. 2023. doi: 10.3390/machines11030381.

9 Multi-Objective Optimization of Hydroxyapatite-added EDM Process for 316L SS in the Context of Biomedical Applications

Md Al-Amin, Ahmad Majdi Abdul-Rani, Iqtidar Ahmed Gul, Adeel Hassan, and Mohd Danish

9.1 INTRODUCTION

316L SS is a surgical-grade material, which is extensively used in fixation device production such as screws, plates, nails, and total hip joints. In the USA, around 70% of hip joints are made of 316L steel. The addition of more chromium in 316L contents not only improved the corrosion resistance by developing a passive oxide layer but also reduced the percentage of nickel content, which causes inflammatory reactions in the body. The demand for 316L steel is showing an upward trend in biomedical industries because of its availability, low cost, ease to manufacture, good biocompatible and corrosion resistance [1–3]. However, the failure of 316L steel-based implant is proposed to be caused by wear, corrosion, fatigue, and bacterial infection in the human body, which are surface-dependent issues [4]. Surface roughness (SR) is an effective factor, which assists to improve the cell's adhesion and protein adsorption on the machined surface resulting in a new tissue born. The proposed optimal SR for an ideal implant ranges from 0.4 to 7.4 μm [1], [5]. Recast layer thickness (RLT) significantly influences the biocompatibility, bio functions and durability of the biomaterials [4, 6] but a thick recast layer may cause mechanical malfunction due to storing stresses and declining compression stress in the coating, which are developed by rapid quenching and melted materials impinging during the machining [1, 7, 8]. Therefore, the obtained thick recast layer should be removed by further polishing process [9, 10]. Hydroxyapatite (HA) is a bio-ceramic powder consisting of

DOI: 10.1201/9781003456018-9

Ca, P, H, and O, which is used to form a biocompatible layer on the modified surface and improve the biological responses of the biomaterials. Nonetheless, it attributes to a high electrical resistivity [1, 11, 12].

The processing of 316L steel is very challenging through the conventional processes such as CNC milling, turning, boring, shaping, CNC lathe, and so on due to its hardness, ductility, and heat resistance behaviour. Besides, the machined surface through these processes cannot ensure biological responses. As a consequence, several coating techniques including electrochemical, plasma spray, sol-gel, and so on are employed to form a coating on shaped 316L steel, which added more cost in the process [2, 5]. Electro-discharge machining (EDM) known as a non-conventional fabrication process is an electrical-thermal process, which can shape and form a coating on the machined part simultaneously retaining a gap between the work-part and tool-electrode. The topography and shape of the machined surface follow the structure and surface condition of the electrode. This process can machine the materials having complex shapes, thin, hard, and brittleness. As a result, the EDM process is successfully utilized in the fabrication of moulds, dies, aerospace parts, and bio-components [2, 13], while a low machining efficiency including a low material removal rate, poor surface integrity with a high roughness, stochastic behaviour during machining and only capable of the conductive materials make negative impacts on EDM applications [11, 14]. To overcome these problems of the EDM process, an innovative process has been introduced in 1980 called the powder mixed-EDM (PM-EDM) technique in which the electrically conductive or semi-conductive particles are mixed in the dielectric liquids to improve the overall system efficiency by ameliorating flushing system, widening plasma channel, and multiple sparks formation. It is assumed that the mechanism of migration and deposition of the fused materials occurs during the PM-EDM process by melting, chemical reactions, and solidification. It has been believed that the addition of electrically conductive powders such as TiC, Al_2O_3, SiC, Al, Cu, Ti, Gr, Si, and so on not only improves the machining performance but also delivers a low SR and RLT with fewer micro-cracks and shallow craters because of enlarging the machining gap, enhancing the flushing system and formation of the multiple ignitions by the single discharge [2, 15, 16].

The goal of this research work is to reduce SR and RLT through HA mixed-EDM process. The second aim of this study is to explore the influence of added powder and associated factors on the responses. The final aim includes acquiring the optimal solutions for the performances. It is hypothesized that the addition of the nano-HA powder in the EDM oil minimizes the SR and RLT by improving flushing performance, enlarging the machining gap and dispersion of the electrical sparks through the gap. However, the overall system efficiency and measures of the machining performances highly rely on EDM process variables that are electrical and non-electrical categories. Optimization of the associated variables is required to obtain the optimal machining responses as the EDM technique shows stochastic behaviour during the machining. In this research work, electrical factors such as peak current, gap voltage, and pulse-on time with a fixed positive polarity and 50% duty cycle were considered. The approaches such as RSM, Taguchi and Grey relational analysis were conducted only for the single objective studies, which were not effective because of the conflicting nature of the obtained results [17, 18]. Thus, this research work used a superior technique called NSGA-II to predict the optimal combinations of the process factors for the best responses considering multiple objectives.

9.2 METHODOLOGY

9.2.1 MATERIALS AND PROCESS

A CNC die-sinker EDM (model: FP60EA; brand: Mitsubishi; country of origin: Japan) was utilized to do machining the workpiece. A separate tank with a capacity of 20 l was used to provide the continuous supply of the powder-mixed EDM oil into the operating tank with a capacity of 200 l. A cutting depth of 0.7 mm was carried out for all of the experiments maintaining an initial gap setting of 0.01 mm between the workpiece and tool-electrode. A positive tool polarity and fixed duty cycle of 50% were chosen for all of the conducted experiments. A schematic model of the PM-EDM technique is presented in Figure 9.1.

A surgical grade 316L austenitic stainless-steel plate of 5 mm × 400 mm × 400 mm purchased from Mechatech Solution, Malaysia was adopted as workpiece material. The as-received plate was cut into small pieces with a size of 5 mm × 9 mm × 10 mm through Wire-cut EDM. Elemental analysis of the purchased 316L steel and the machined surface is reported in Figure 9.2a,b. Commercially pure titanium was chosen as the tool-electrode material because of having biocompatibility and low erosion rate [19]. The purchased pure titanium was sliced with a size of 85 mm × 9.5 mm × 10.5 mm using Wire-cut EDM as well. Nano-size HA powder with a size of 40 nm purchased from Mechatech Solution, Malaysia was adopted as the additive powder as per the design of experiments.

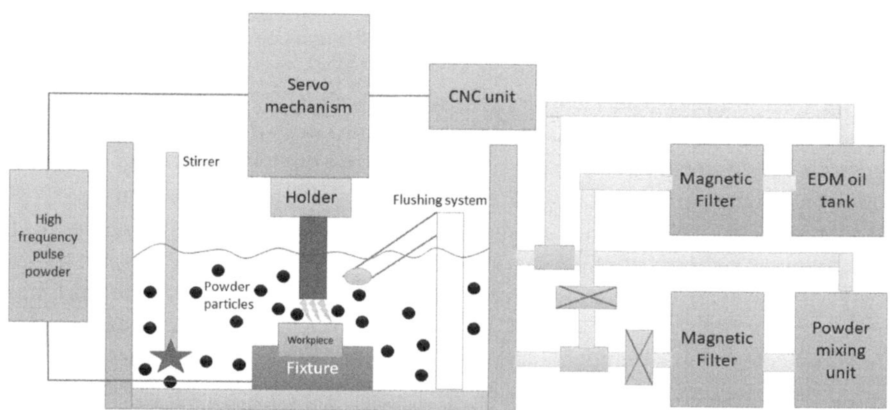

FIGURE 9.1 Schematic model of the PM-EDM technique.

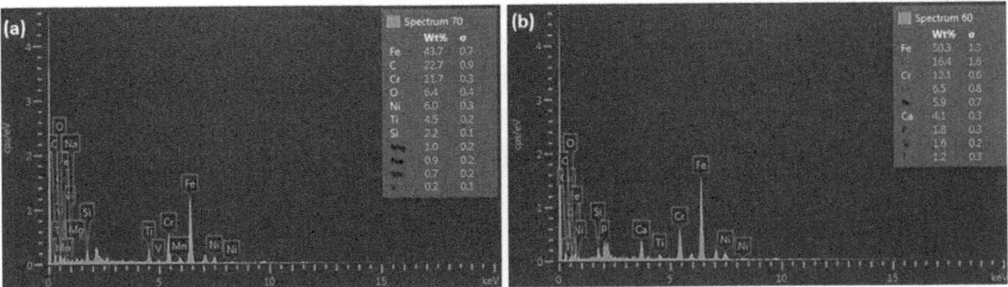

FIGURE 9.2 Elemental analysis using energy-dispersive X-ray for (a) Purchased 316L steel, (b) machined 316L steel.

TABLE 9.1
Selected variables and their levels

Machining factors	Units	Levels			Responses	Unit
Peak current (A)	A	5	7	10	SR	μm
Pulse-on time (B)	μs	8	12	16	RLT	μm
HA amount (C)	g/l	7	10	15		
Gap voltage (D)	V	150	220	260		

9.2.2 Experimental Design Using the Taguchi Approach

Taguchi-based orthogonal array L9 (3^4) was performed using Minitab 19 software to minimize the run of experiments, which reduced the experimental cost and time. Mathematical modelling, ANOVA analysis, and effects of the factors on the responses were conducted through Minitab 19 software as well. The process factors such as peak current (A), pulse-on time (μs), HAp amount (g/l), and gap voltage (V) were considered for this research. The selected variables with their levels are reported in Table 9.1.

Here, the minimizing responses were preferred for both SR and RLT. The signal-to-noise ratio (S/N) as a quality loss function was calculated using the given mathematical equation (9.1).

(i) Minimum-the-better

$$S/N = -\log\left[1/n\sum_{i=1}^{n} y^{\wedge}2\right] \tag{9.1}$$

where: y represents the nth observations of SR and RLT.

The nonlinear with the first-order mathematical model was generated and given in Equation (9.2)

$$Y = \beta_o + \sum_{i=1}^{n} \beta i X i + \sum_{i<}^{n} \sum_{j=2}^{n} \beta i j X i X j + \alpha \qquad (9.2)$$

where: Y is the response, β is the regression coefficient, n is the number of independent variables (process factor), X denotes independent variables, and α gives an error value.

9.2.3 MEASUREMENT OF THE PERFORMANCES

A profilometer (Brand: Mitutoyo; Model: SV3000; Origin: Japan) was used to calculate SR. The measurement of SR was conducted following the standard of ISO 3274:1996. The average roughness (Ra) was carried out for the modified surfaces selecting a measurement length of 8 mm.

The coated 316L steel samples were mounted by a mounting press machine (Model: Simplimet@1000; Origin: USA). The mounted specimens were polished using a grinder-polisher machine (Model: Metaserv250) with 400, 600, 800, 1200, and 1500 grits SiC grinding papers. The polished specimens were immersed into the prepared Carpenters etchant solution ($FeCl_3$: 8.5 g; Ethanol: 122 ml; Hydrochloric acid: 122 ml; $CuCl_2$: 2.4 g; Nitric acid: 6 ml) for 3 s to remove the debris and burrs. The polished and etched specimens were investigated to measure RLT through a scanning electron microscope (SEM) (Model: Zeiss Evo LS15; Origin: Germany) applying an EHT powder supply of 20 KV and magnification from 500 to 3.00Kx.

9.2.4 DETAILS OF NSGA-II

Multi-objective optimization of the process factors was performed using NSGA-II which is comprehensively used rather than the other MOGA approaches. The Pareto

---

TABLE 9.2

Parameters setting for conducting NSGA-II

Selected parameters	Measurement
Population mode	Double vector
Population size	300
Selection	Tournament
Crossover percentages	0.9
Crossover mode	Intermediate
Crossover ratio	1
Mutation	Constraint dependent
Pareto fraction	0.6
Migration	Forward
Migration fraction	0.1

optimal fronts for the multi-objectives were obtained using MATLAB software [20]. The parameter settings for conducting NSGA-II are shown in Table 9.2.

9.3 RESULTS AND DISCUSSION

This section discusses the experimental data acquired from conducting nine experiments using L9 (3^4) orthogonal array and analysis of data. Table 9.3 shows the L9 experimental design with results and S/N ratio for the responses.

9.3.1 SIGNAL-TO-NOISE (S/N) ANALYSIS FOR THE RESPONSES

The function of quality loss, which is a continuous function explains the deviation of a design factor from the absolute value and a larger S/N value provides the desired combination of the process factors for the optimal response [21]. Since minimal SR and RLT were the desired mode, the lower-the-better were considered for SR and RLT. From Table 9.3, run_1 reveals the highest S/N ratio values for SR and RLT.

9.3.2 ANALYSIS OF THE MAIN EFFECTS PLOTS

From the main effects plots of the responses shown in Figure 9.3a,b, it is noticed that the peak current, HA amount, and pulse-on time are treated as the influential factors for SR and RLT, whereas the gap voltage shows a negative trend for the responses The most significant factor for the performances is the peak current accompanied by the pulse-on time and HA amount but the HA amount shows an exceptional trend for SR. As shown in Figure 9.3a,b, minimum SR is predicted when the peak current is 5 A, pulse-on time is 8 µs, HA amount is 15 g/l, and gap voltage is 260 V. In addition, minimum RLT is obtained when the peak current is 5 A, pulse-on time is 8 µs, HA amount is 7 g/l, and gap voltage is 260 V.

TABLE 9.3
L9 experimental design and values of responses

	Process factors				Responses			
Run	A (A)	B (µs)	C (g/l)	D (V)	SR (µm)	S/N for SR	RLT (µm)	S/N ratio for RLT
1	5	8	10	260	2.039	-6.18834	6.1	-15.7065967
2	5	12	15	150	2.572	-8.20542	9.22	-19.2946184
3	5	16	7	220	3.565	-11.0412	8.4366	-18.5233492
4	7	8	15	220	2.7	-8.62728	8.8533	-18.9421036
5	7	12	7	260	3.875	-11.7654	9.038	-19.1214467
6	7	16	10	150	3.828	-11.6594	11.05	-20.8672456
7	10	8	7	150	4.32	-12.7097	9.711	-19.7452791
8	10	12	10	220	3.94	-11.9099	12.8	-22.1441994
9	10	16	15	260	4.135	-12.3295	15.895	-24.0252106

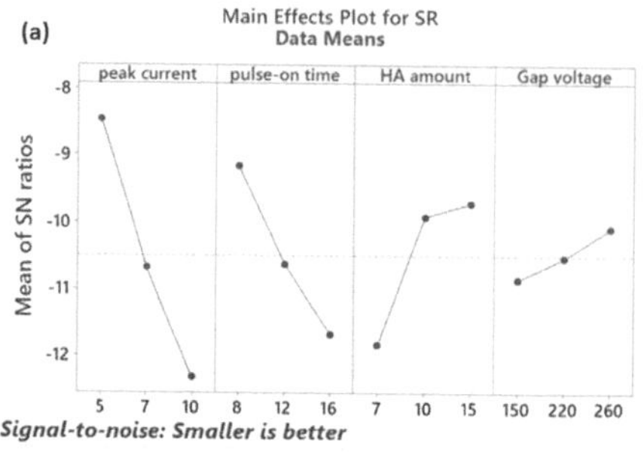

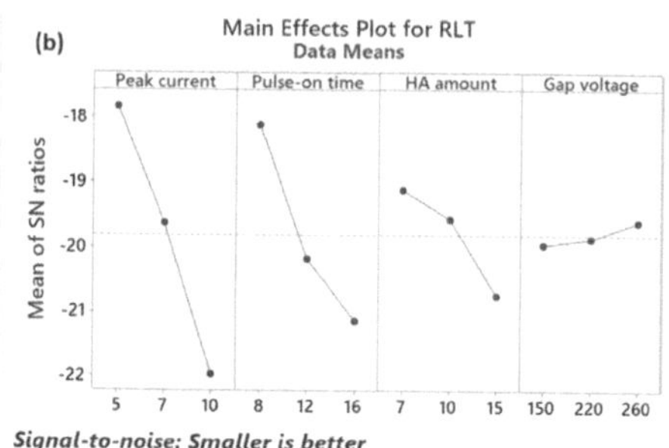

FIGURE 9.3 Main effects plots for SR and RLT.

TABLE 9.4
Summary of ANOVA results for SR and RLT

Responses	Factors with p-value				Model accuracy		Contribution			
	A	**B**	**C**	**D**	**R-sq (%)**	**R-sq (adj%)**	**A (%)**	**B (%)**	**C (%)**	**D (%)**
SR (µm)	0.004	0.023	0.033	0.37	95.35	92.56	56.68	19.82	15.75	1.57
RLT (µm)	0.0001	0.0001	0.001	0.29	99.35	98.66	57.19	29.84	12.07	0.24

	SR	**RLT**
Regression model	0.001	0.0001

9.3.3 Analysis of SR Outputs

The ANOVA results for SR was given in Table 9.4. From Table 9.4, the p-value for the regression pattern is lower than 0.05, which indicates the statistical significance of the model [14]. The data of R-sq and R-sq (adj) are 95.35% and 92.56%, respectively, which confirms the regression model offering robust analysis of the interactions between the process parameters and SR. The variables such as peak current, pulse-on time, and HA amount are manifested to be statistically momentous as the p values are lower than 0.05. The variables such as A, B, and C contribute to SR by 56.68%, 19.82%, and 15.75%, respectively, while machining the 316L steel.

A general form of non-linear mathematical model for SR was developed for conducting the multi-objective optimization, which is given as follows:

$$SR = -0.6 + 0.612*A + 0.155*B + 0.013*C - 0.0055*D$$
$$- 0.0203*A*B - 0.0108*A*C + 0.00052*B*D.$$

A contour plot offers a 2D presentation in which all points with the same responses are joined to create a constant response contour line [17]. The combined effects of the process variables on SR are represented in Figure 9.4a–c.

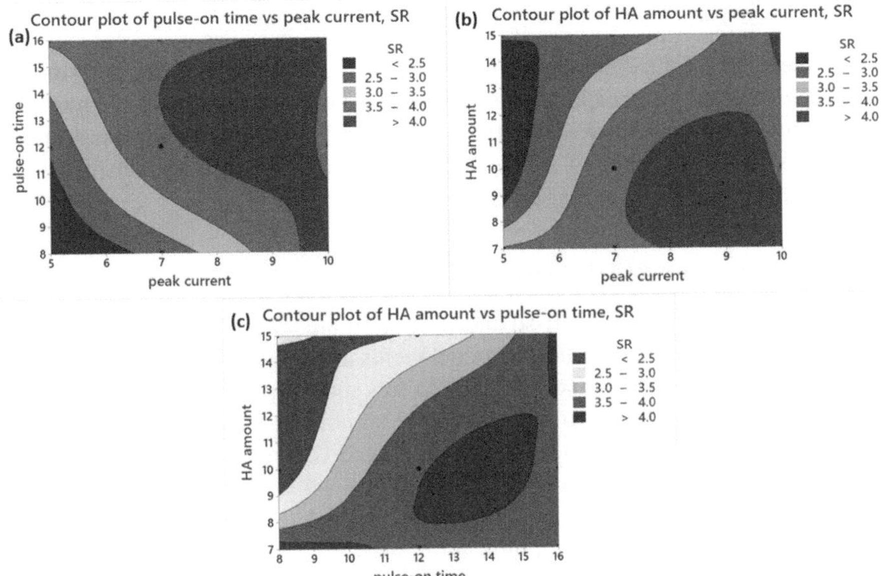

FIGURE 9.4 Contour plots for SR (a) B vs A, (b) C vs A, (c) C vs B.

From the contour plot shown in Figure 9.4a, the lowest values of SR are observed at the peak current ranging from 5 to 6.5 A and pulse-on time varied from 8 to 11.5 µs, while SR reveals the highest values when the peak current and pulse-on time increase from 7 to 10 A and from 8 to 16 µs, respectively. SR increases from 2.5 to 4 µm while improving the peak current from 6.5 to 9.5 A with the pulse-on time ranging from 8 to 16 µs. In Figure 9.4b, at the lowest peak current values and HA amount ranging from 8.6 to 14.8 g/l, SR discloses the lowest values that are located in dark blue colour. Further increment of peak current up to 10 A with all the HA amount (from 7 to 15 g/l) results from an augment of SR ranging from 2.5 to 4 µm. The dark green zone highlights the maximum fitted values of SR corresponding to the peak current ranging from 7.3 to 10 A with the HA amount varied from 7 to 11.8 g/l and 13.5 to 15 g/l. As shown in Figure 9.4c, SR shows the lowest values for the pulse-on time values from 8 to 11.5 µs and the HA amount ranged from 9 to 15 g/l is positioned in dark red colour. Further increment of pulse-on time up to 16 µs with all the HA amount causes a rise in SR varied from 2.5 to 4 µm. The areas that represent SR of more than 4 µm are marked by the purple colour.

From the above analyses, it is apparent that with increasing the peak current and pulse-on time, SR increases due to the application of additional electric sparks in the plasma channel, which produce wide and deep craters with a single discharge resulting in a rough machined surface. It is noted that the addition of a small quantity of 7 g/l HA powder in the EDM oil offers a rougher surface compared to more than 7 g/l HA particle application because of the rapid settling tendency of the HA particles. The availability of HA particles in the machining gap is low as a result of rapid settling causing minimal spark dispersion. As the HA has very little electrical conductivity, initially it tends the electrodes to come closer to each other resulting in a poor flushing system and abnormal sparks formation. Due to abnormal sparks production, large craters are produced and a few nanoparticles and debris are stuck on the electrode surface, which form the craters on the machined surface similar to the shape of them. Further increment of the HA powder concentration up to 15 g/l leads to lowering the electrical resistivity of the EDM oil due to chain-like formation resulting in an enlargement of the discharge gap, which enhances the flushing system and creates the shallow craters [2, 16].

9.3.4 ANALYSIS OF RLT OUTPUTS

From Table 9.4, the values of R-sq and R-sq (adj) are 99.35% and 98.66%, respectively, which indicates the regression model yields a strong analysis of the interactions between the process factors and RLT. The factors such as peak current, pulse-on time, and HA amount are shown to be statistically significant since p values are smaller than 0.05. The process variables such as A, B, and C contribute to RLT by 57.19%, 29.84%, and 12.07%, respectively.

A general form of non-linear mathematical model for SR was developed for conducting the multi-objective optimization, which is given as follows:

$$RLT = -12.88 + 1.201*A + 1.08*B + 0.695*C - 0.0031*D$$
$$+ 0.0341*A*B\ 0.0621*A*C + 0.000791*B*D.$$

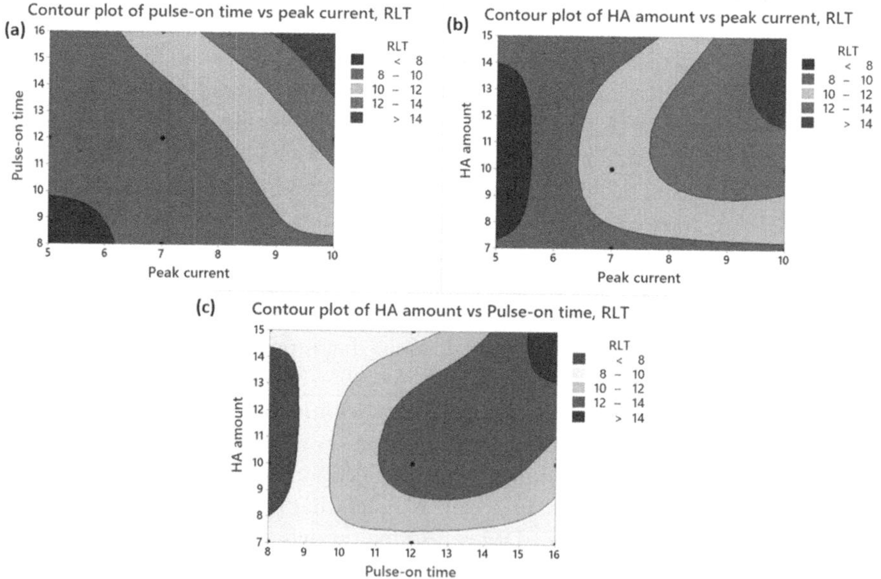

FIGURE 9.5 Contour plots for RLT (a) B vs A, (b) C vs A, (c) C vs B.

The combined effects of the process factors on RLT were represented in Figure 9.5a–c. From the contour plot shown in Figure 9.5a, at the lowest values of both peak current and pulse-on time, RLT shows the lowest values that are located in dark blue colour. Further, an increase of peak current up to 10 A with the pulse-on time (from 9.8 to 16 µs) results from an improvement of RLT ranging from 8 to 14 µm. The dark green zone indicates the maximum fitted values of RLT for higher both peak current and pulse-on time. In Figure 9.5b, the smallest values of RLT (dark blue area) are remarked at the lowest peak current values and HA amount varied from 7.4 to 13.8 g/l, whereas RLT displays the highest values (dark green area) when the peak current reaches the maximum values and HA amount increases from 11.5 to 15 g/l. RLT increases from 8 to 14 µm due to augmenting the peak current from 5 to 10 A with all HA amount values. In Figure 9.5c, RLT shows the lowest values for the lowest pulse-on time values with the HA amount ranging from 8 to 13.5 g/l which is highlighted by dark red colour. Further increment of pulse-on time with all HA amount values causes an ascent in RLT varied from 8 to 14 µm. RLT shows the maximum where the combination of pulse-on time and HA amount is the maximum that is located in purple colour.

From this section, it is concluded that RLT increases with raising the peak current, HA amount, and pulse-on time during machining. Increment of the peak current and pulse-on time yield exceeding electrical energy in the plasma channel converted into heat energy, which results in more decomposition of the electrode materials, added HA particles, and EDM oil. These melted materials improve the recast layer formation. Figure 9.2b confirms the migration of the melted material on the machined part. Besides, an increment of HA amount ensures more HA particles are present in the machining gap creating the chain-like formation due to a field emission and a capacitive effect, which assists to get deposited on the machined surface forming a thick recast layer [12]. The measured RLT show comparatively thinner than the RLT achieved by Chander et.al. (2017), Abdul Azeez et.al. (2019), and Chander et.al. (2018) using the same amount of HA powders addition (15 g/l), which can eliminate the further polishing process [10]. A thick recast layer contains more residual stresses and reduces the compression stress resulting in the mechanical failure of the machined devices [8] while a thin recast layer is expected for long time application.

9.3.5 MULTI-OBJECTIVE OPTIMIZATION THROUGH NSGA-II

From the experimental point of view, the selected responses such as SR and RLT increase when metal erosion increases. However, from the manufacturing point of view, SR and RLT are chosen as the "Smallest the better". It is very challenging to find out the proper combinations of the associated factors that offer larger metal erosion with smaller RLT and SR. In the present study, two objectives have been followed that are given as follows:

Objective (1): Minimum (RLT)
Objective (2): Minimum (SR).

The Pareto optimal frontier that shows the optimal sets of solutions considering the objectives is depicted in Figure 9.6. Among the 120 non-dominated solutions, the best

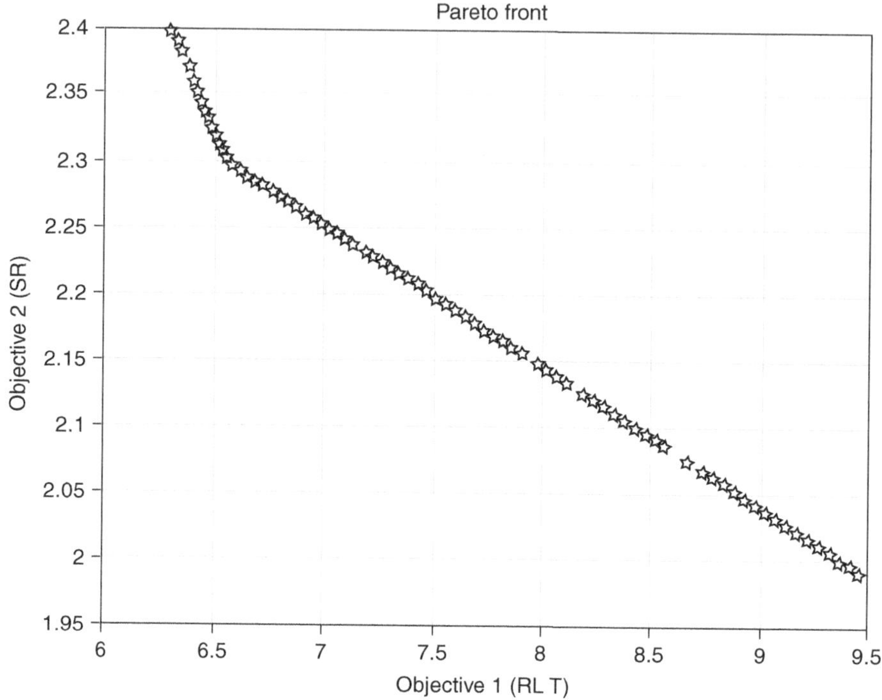

FIGURE 9.6 Optimal Pareto frontiers.

TABLE 9.5
The best seven optimal solutions for SR and RLT

					Predicted results	
Sl. no	A (A)	B (µs)	C (g/l)	D (V)	RLT	SR
1	5	8	7	199	6.47	2.333
2	5	8	7.25	224.6	6.641	2.29
3	5	8	14.45	224.65	9.423	1.996
4	5	8	9.63	224.6	7.56	2.193
5	5	8	11	224.68	8.086	2.137
6	5	8	9	224.7	7.349	2.215
7	5	8	10.36	224.4	7.84	2.163

seven solutions (predicted results) were selected corresponding to the process factors that were reported in Table 9.5. In Figure 9.6, RLT and SR show a conflicting relation. Increasing RLT leads to a decrease in SR. A rise in RLT from 6.47 to 9.423 µm is demonstrated, whereas a decrease in SR from 2.33 to 1.996 µm is shown.

From Table 9.5, the errors for RLT and SR were reported below 10%, which guaranteed excellent prediction of the combination of process factors for RLT and SR.

Solution no.1 revealed the smallest errors for both responses. The lowest RLT and highest SR of 6.47 and 2.33 µm, respectively, were obtained at a peak current of 5 A, pulse-on time of 8 µs, HA amount of 7 g/l, and gap voltage of 199 V, whereas the highest RLT and lowest SR of 9.423 and 1.996 µm, respectively, were calculated at a 5 A peak current, 8 µs pulse-on time, 14.45 g/l HA amount, and 224.65 V gap voltage. It is seen that a high HA amount was also suggested for increasing RLT and decreasing SR. The best-fitted solutions for minimizing both RLT and SR may be chosen from solutions no. 1 to 7.

9.4 CONCLUSIONS

From the present research, the following conclusions can be included:

1. Gap voltage has been regarded as a non-significant factor for SR and RLT although the peak current followed by the pulse-on time, and HA amount is the most critical factor for the performances. The HA amount revealed the largest contribution (15.75%) to SR followed by 12.07% to RLT. SR raises with the improvement of peak current and pulse-on time but a rise in the HA amount in the EDM oil encourages a low SR. Moreover, a high peak current, pulse-on time, and HA amount cause a high RLT. The smallest SR and RLT of 2.039 and 6.1 µm, respectively, are measured for a 5 A peak current, 8 µs pulse-on time, and 10 g/l HA amount while the largest RLT of 6.1 µm is calculated at the peak current of 10 A, pulse-on time of 16 µs, and HA amount of 15 g/l. Furthermore, the biggest SR is observed while employing 10 A peak current, 8 µs pulse-on time, and 7 g/l HA amount.
2. Through the multi-objective optimization approach, the best combinations of the related process variables for the optimal outputs that are conflicting in nature have been achieved. The best 120 solutions according to the objectives have been acquired from which anyone can be chosen based on the requirement of the process engineer or new researcher. The required low SR and RLT are predicted for the combinations of 5 A peak current, 8 µs pulse-on time, 14.9 g/l HA amount, and 260 V gap voltage.

This research work is expected to provide an effective approach to the process engineers or new researchers for manufacturing biomedical devices made of 316L steel. A uniform and thin recast layer with the micro-cracks free and nanopores surface is confirmed using SEM analysis that is intended to eliminate the failure of the bio-implant after implantation. Moreover, the obtained thin recast layer may reduce the process of further polishing. The obtained SR ranged from 2.039 to 4.32 µm lies within the optimal range (0.4–7.4 µm) for biomedical applications.

ACKNOWLEDGMENTS

The authors reveal their cordial gratefulness and admiration to Universiti Teknologi Petronas (UTP) for providing components and working place. The present research was fully assisted by the ministry of higher education, Malaysia through FRGS grant: (FRGS/1/2020/TK0/UTP/02/39).

REFERENCES

[1] M. Al-Amin, A. M. Abdul Rani, A. A. Abdu Aliyu, M. A. Abdul Razak, S. Hastuty, and M. G. Bryant, "Powder mixed-EDM for potential biomedical applications: A critical review," *Mater. Manuf. Process.*, pp. 1789–1811, 2020, doi: 10.1080/10426914.2020.1779939.

[2] M. Al-Amin *et al.*, "Assessment of PM-EDM cycle factors influence on machining responses and surface properties of biomaterials: A comprehensive review," *Precis. Eng.*, 2020.

[3] T. M. Abdel-Fattah, D. Loftis, and A. Mahapatro, "Nanosized controlled surface pretreatment of biometallic alloy 316L stainless steel," *J. Biomed. Nanotechnol.*, vol. 7, no. 6, pp. 794–800, 2011.

[4] J. D. Majumdar, A. Kumar, S. Pityana, and I. Manna, "Laser surface melting of AISI 316L stainless steel for bio-implant application," *Proc. Natl. Acad. Sci. India Sect. A Phys. Sci.*, vol. 88, no. 3, pp. 387–403, 2018.

[5] C. Prakash, H. K. Kansal, B. S. Pabla, S. Puri, and A. Aggarwal, "Electric discharge machining – A potential choice for surface modification of metallic implants for orthopedic applications: A review," *Proc. Inst. Mech. Eng. Part B J. Eng. Manuf.*, vol. 230, no. 2, pp. 331–353, 2016, doi: 10.1177/0954405415579113.

[6] N. Eliaz, "Corrosion of metallic biomaterials: A review," *Materials (Basel).*, vol. 12, no. 3, p. 407, 2019.

[7] B. Singh, G. Singh, B. S. Sidhu, and N. Bhatia, "In-vitro assessment of HA-Nb coating on Mg alloy ZK60 for biomedical applications," *Mater. Chem. Phys.*, vol. 231, pp. 138–149, 2019.

[8] S. S. Joshi, S. Katakam, H. Singh Arora, S. Mukherjee, and N. B. Dahotre, "Amorphous coatings and surfaces on structural materials," *Crit. Rev. Solid State Mater. Sci.*, vol. 41, no. 1, pp. 1–46, 2016.

[9] R. Singh, S. Schruefer, S. Wilson, J. Gibmeier, and R. Vassen, "Influence of coating thickness on residual stress and adhesion-strength of cold-sprayed Inconel 718 coatings," *Surf. coatings Technol.*, vol. 350, pp. 64–73, 2018.

[10] A. A. Aliyu *et al.*, "A review of additive mixed-electric discharge machining: current status and future perspectives for surface modification of biomedical implants," *Adv. Mater. Sci. Eng.*, vol. 2017, 2017, doi: 10.1155/2017/8723239.

[11] M. Al-Amin, A. M. Abdul Rani, A. A. Abdu Aliyu, M. G. Bryant, M. Danish, and A. Ahmad, "Bio-ceramic coatings adhesion and roughness of biomaterials through PM-EDM: a comprehensive review," *Mater. Manuf. Process.*, vol. 00, no. 00, pp. 1157–1180, 2020, doi: 10.1080/10426914.2020.1772483.

[12] M. Al-Amin *et al.*, "Investigation of machining and modified surface features of 316L steel through novel hybrid of HA/CNT added-EDM process," *Mater. Chem. Phys.*, p. 125320, 2021.

[13] M. Kunieda, B. Lauwers, K. P. Rajurkar, and B. M. Schumacher, "Advancing EDM through fundamental insight into the process," *CIRP Ann.*, vol. 54, no. 2, pp. 64–87, 2005.

[14] M. Hanif, A. Wasim, A. H. Shah, S. Noor, M. Sajid, and N. Mujtaba, "Optimization of process parameters using graphene-based dielectric in electric discharge machining of AISI D2 steel," *Int. J. Adv. Manuf. Technol.*, vol. 103, no. 9, pp. 3735–3749, 2019.

[15] P. Pecas and E. Henriques, "Influence of silicon powder-mixed dielectric on conventional electrical discharge machining," *Int. J. Mach. Tools Manuf.*, vol. 43, no. 14, pp. 1465–1471, 2003.

[16] G. Talla, S. Gangopadhayay, and C. K. Biswas, "State of the art in powder-mixed electric discharge machining: A review," *Proc. Inst. Mech. Eng. Part B J. Eng. Manuf.*, vol. 231, no. 14, pp. 2511–2526, 2017, doi: 10.1177/0954405416634265.

[17] R. Magabe, N. Sharma, K. Gupta, and J. P. Davim, "Modeling and optimization of Wire-EDM parameters for machining of Ni 55.8 Ti shape memory alloy using hybrid approach of Taguchi and NSGA-II," *Int. J. Adv. Manuf. Technol.*, vol. 102, no. 5, pp. 1703–1717, 2019.

[18] K. Kumar, V. Singh, P. Katyal, and N. Sharma, "EDM -drilling in Ti-6Al-7Nb: experimental investigation and optimization using NSGA-II," *Int. J. Adv. Manuf. Technol.*, vol. 104, no. 5, pp. 2727–2738, 2019.

[19] M. Niinomi, "Recent titanium R&D for biomedical applications in Japan," *Jom*, vol. 51, no. 6, pp. 32–34, 1999.

[20] M. Al-Amin, A. M. Abdul-Rani, R. Ahmed, and T. V. V. L. N. Rao, "Multiple-objective optimization of hydroxyapatite-added EDM technique for processing of 316L-steel," *Mater. Manuf. Process.*, vol. 36, no. 10, pp. 1134–1145, 2021, doi: 10.1080/10426914.2021.1885715.

[21] E. Kuram and B. Ozcelik, "Multi-objective optimization using Taguchi based grey relational analysis for micro-milling of Al 7075 material with ball nose end mill," *Measurement*, vol. 46, no. 6, pp. 1849–1864, 2013.

Index